Helpful herbs for health and beauty

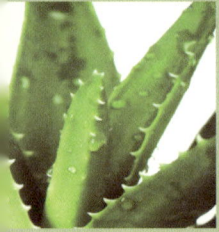

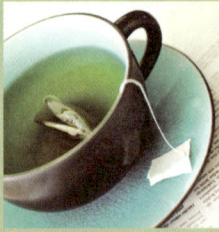

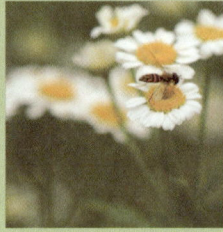

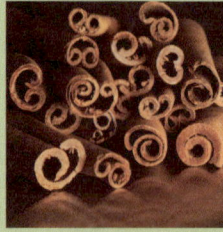

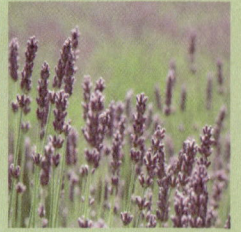

Helpful
HERBS
for health
and beauty

Look and feel great, naturally

Barbara Griggs

brilliantideas

CAREFUL NOW

Treat herbs with respect and use them carefully and all should be well. You can find details of how to contact a qualified herbalist in the Resources section, and remember that you will also need medical advice sometimes. This book is not a substitute for advice from your own doctor and/or herbal specialist, though there are many minor ailments which can be easily treated with home doctoring.

If you're taking prescription drugs don't take herbal medicines at the same time without professional advice, either from a fully qualified herbalist or from your doctor. Always tell your doctor if you are taking herbal medicines, as some can interact with prescription drugs. If you are pregnant or breastfeeding, only use herbs in culinary quantities – don't, for instance, drink gallons of peppermint tea. Never, ever take anything internally that is meant to be applied externally and don't use undiluted essential oils, except for tea tree and lavender. Always keep them where children can't get at them.

Though every effort has been made to provide up-to-date, accurate information, neither the author nor the publisher can be held responsible or liable for any loss or claim arising out of the suggestions made in this book. Everyone is different and we don't know your specific circumstances. Be sensible and careful and, if in doubt, always seek specific advice.

Website addresses were checked at the time of going to press, but may change over time so neither publisher nor author can guarantee the availability or content of these sites.

First published in 2008 by
The Infinite Ideas Company Limited
36 St Giles
Oxford
OX1 3LD
United Kingdom
www.infideas.com

A CIP catalogue record for this book is available from the British Library

ISBN 978-1-904902-42-3

Designed and typeset by Baseline Arts Ltd, Oxford
Printed in India

Brilliant ideas

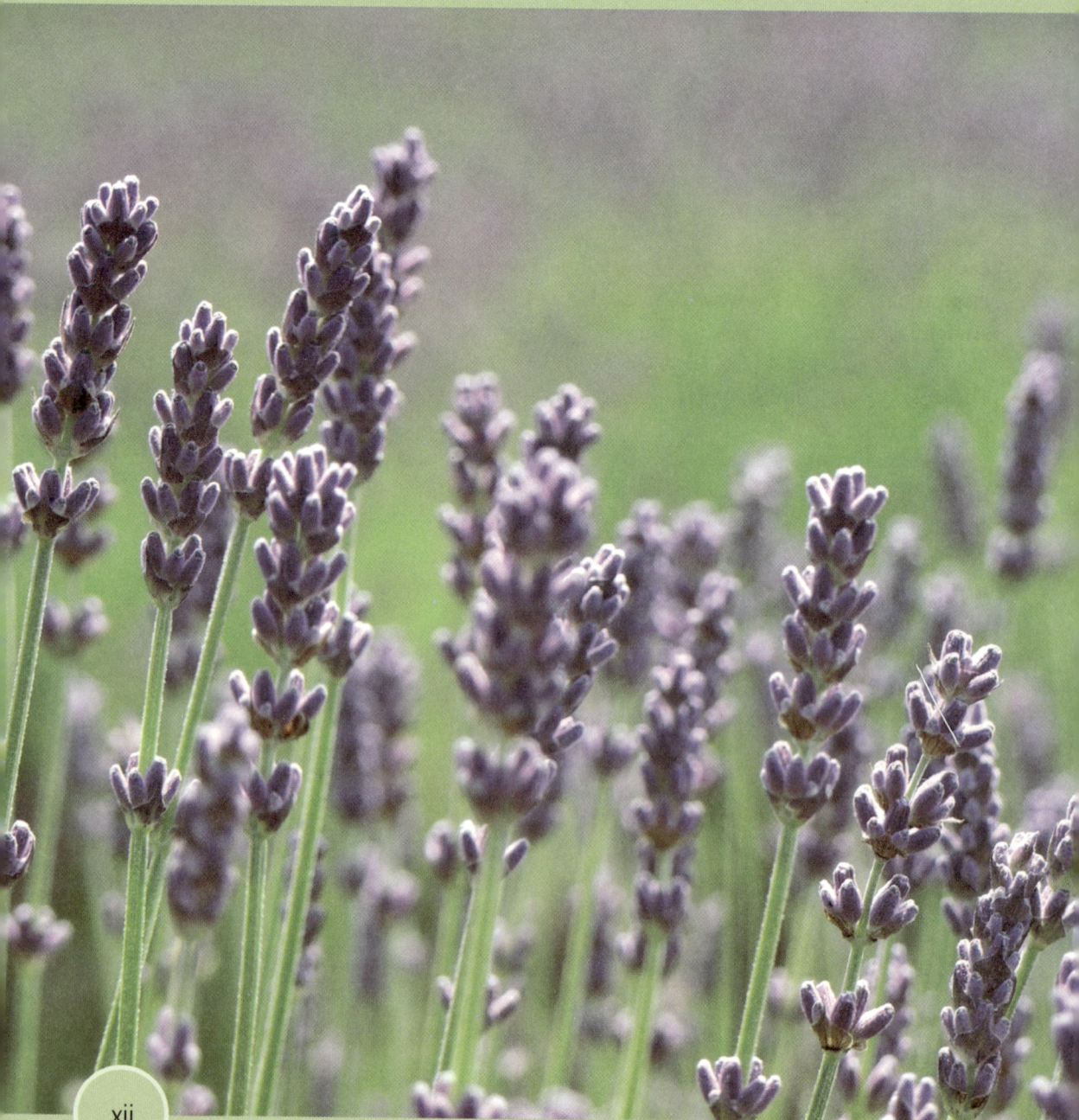

Brilliant features

Each chapter of this book is designed to provide you with an inspirational idea that you can read quickly and put into practice straight away.

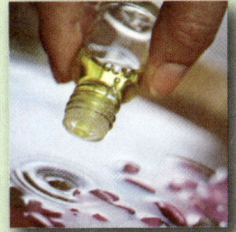

Throughout you'll find three features that will help you to get right to the heart of the idea:

- *Here's an idea for you* Take it on board and give it a go – right here, right now. Get an idea of how well you're doing so far.

- *Defining idea* Words of wisdom from masters and mistresses of the art, plus some interesting hangers-on.

- *How did it go?* If at first you do succeed, try to hide your amazement. If, on the other hand, you don't, then this is where you'll find a Q and A that highlights common problems and how to get over them.

Introduction

Is there a future for old-fashioned herbal medicine? With all the wonders of modern medicine at our disposal, why should we still bother with herbs? What can they do that a prescription drug can't fix – and faster too?

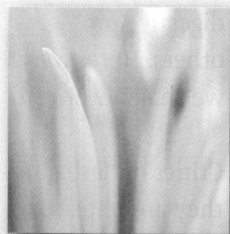

These are questions that sceptics ask. But I firmly believe that herbal and modern medicine can work side by side to give us the best of both worlds.

There is no herbal substitute for the skills of the surgeon and the anaesthetist, for the technological marvels on which modern medicine often depends for diagnosis or treatment, for the knowledge and experience of doctors, and for the many brilliant drugs – steroids, antibacterials, antifungals, antiparasitics, antiepileptics, drugs to combat cancer, major antidepressants, antihistamines – developed over decades by the pharmaceutical industry.

But, equally, herbs have properties for which there is no equivalent in the world of synthetic drugs. They can boost the body's own cleansing and detoxing activity. They can calm nerves on edge, and help balance out-of-whack hormones. They can clear a foggy brain or slow a racing irregular heartbeat. They can promote healing and give healthful sleep with no drug-induced hangover. They can be fabulous friends at times of stress or exhaustion or anxiety. And, properly used, they can do all this with few or none of the side effects which are the bane of so many drugs.

They can be especially useful in those many disorders where conventional medicine seems to have run out of ideas beyond yet another exciting new drug – things like digestive problems, arthritis, eczema, acne, asthma and chronic bronchitis, among others. Herbs are also, quite literally, 'green medicine'. We may run out of oil, but we shall never run out of healing plants.

Critics of herbal medicine tend to suggest either that herbs are ineffectual or that they are untested and therefore dangerous. It's true that most of the remedies we use today evolved slowly over long centuries, and were discovered and developed by ordinary people beyond the reach of professional medicine, doctoring their ailments with leaves, flowers, roots and bark from the trees and plants they found in their own patch of countryside. But when some of these 'cures' began to be submitted to searching clinical examination in the late twentieth century, they came through with enhanced reputations. Among them are hawthorn to reinvigorate the heart, devil's claw for arthritis, milk thistle to protect the liver, St John's wort for minor states of depression, including the sun-hungry victims of seasonal affective disorder, and *Ginkgo biloba* for the protection of the ageing brain.

Dozens of other useful herbs have never undergone the rigorous testing of a modern synthetic drug. But centuries of successful use, by professional physicians as well as village wisewomen or busy housewives, will strike most people as perhaps even more satisfactory evidence of their value than five to ten years of clinical testing.

Certainly herbs must be used with caution and respect. Beginners should start with the gentlest and safest of herbs, or get to know what wonders ordinary kitchen herbs and spices – sage, ginger, cayenne, mint – can perform. But as you grow to appreciate herbs, you will gradually become more experienced in their use.

Home doctoring with herbs can be fine for minor ailments. For more serious trouble, you must, of course, see your doctor. But I hope you will also learn to consult a qualified medical herbalist in cases where you feel modern medicine isn't doing as much for you as you would wish – you can track one down through the Resources section. Herbalists are used to working alongside doctors, and if you are taking prescription drugs they will know what herbs can safely be prescribed at the same time. With their long experience and knowledge, they can often clear up problems that may have been bothering you for weeks or months. They will take a long and thorough medical history before they prescribe and can fine-tune a herbal prescription to take into account the whole you with all its problems, not just the bit that's bothering you. This book is no substitute for the knowledge and experience they can offer.

There is still much you can do for yourself if no herbalist is available. And for what the French call the 'little miseries' of life – hangovers, colds, minor burns, a bad tummy upset, odd aches and pains – I'd trust my herbal medicine kit to help fix the problem sooner than any modern drug.

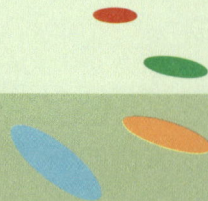

1

Getting started

Welcome to the wonderful world of herbs.

The more you discover about these people-friendly remedies, the more you'll want to explore, experiment and discover.

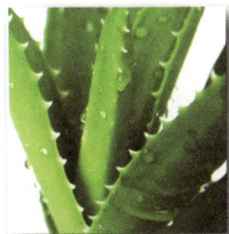

How do you get started? Begin by experimenting with some specially safe and effective herbs for self-doctoring: peppermint tea for indigestion, aloe vera gel for sunburn, an infusion of sage to gargle for a sore throat, a dozen drops of the essential oil of lavender in a bedtime bath to help you wind down and sleep. The more you use herbs, the more confident you will become, and the more you'll want to get to know them.

Just how safe are herbal remedies? Many are actually food medicines, used freely to season food all over the world: thyme, rosemary, sage, lemon balm and garlic from the herb garden, or cinnamon, caraway, ginger, turmeric and cayenne from the spice rack. Numbers of common wildflowers and weeds – nettles, dandelion, cleavers, plantain, meadowsweet, burdock – are actually among the most valuable agents at a herbalist's disposal and are in common and everyday use. If any of these presented a real danger to consumers, you feel that somebody just might have picked up on the fact before now. Where a herb demands special caution in its use, however, I note the fact.

Here's an idea for you...

This is an excellent one for beginners. Propolis, the 'glue' which bonds and protects beehives, is produced by bees from antiseptic resins they harvest from certain trees. Tincture of propolis is one of the most useful items you could have in your medicine cupboard, especially for problems around the mouth, gums and throat. Next time you have a mouth ulcer or a cold sore, apply a few drops of neat propolis on a cotton-wool bud. Gargle with a few drops of propolis in a little warm water for a sore throat, and use a propolis toothpaste to ward off tooth and gum infections.

Nonetheless, as with any therapy, you need to go very carefully, especially if you are a beginner. Pregnant or breastfeeding women should avoid all herbal medicines, and that can even mean food medicines too, apart from normal culinary use. If you are taking prescription drugs, don't take herbal medicines too without the say-so of your doctor: it's possible they may interact and cause a problem.

Don't expect herbs to work miracles. If you're run down from lack of fresh air and exercise, or not enough relaxation and sleep, or if your health is being steadily undermined by a daily diet of junk or heavily processed food, the most skilfully prescribed herbal medicine in the world won't be able to fix things for you.

There is no known herb – or foodstuff, for that matter – to which somebody, somewhere has not had an allergic reaction, minor or major. Be sensible. When you use a 'new' herb topically, patch-test it on your skin. If you're swallowing the stuff, watch out for odd reactions.

Essential oils need to be treated with the utmost respect. Don't take them internally. Never apply them undiluted to the skin: the only exceptions are lavender or tea tree. And by all means use herbs to treat minor ailments such as coughs, sunburn, an upset tummy, a chesty cold. But if symptoms persist or become more severe – go and see your doctor.

In what form should you use herbs? You can make up some herbal remedies yourself: simple infusions of plants such as sage, fresh lemon balm, chamomile or nettle, to be drunk as teas. Most of the herbal remedies you buy in health-food stores or from herbal suppliers come in one of five forms: tinctures, when the healing virtues of the herb are extracted in alcohol; creams and ointments for topical use; made-up pills and capsules; essential oils; and – an ever-swelling number – tea bags. Buy your herbs from a reliable supplier, and carefully observe the maker's dosage instructions, together with any cautions. There are some excellent suppliers online.

'I should certainly not have such confidence in plants to protect me from illness had I not proved to myself the beneficial virtues of dozens of medicinal herbs which, as I have learned during these last years, are commonly employed by country folk.'
JEAN PALAISEUL, *Grandmother's Secrets*

Defining idea…

Be picky when buying herbs. You won't find Gordon Ramsay buying beefsteaks, salmon or olive oil from the cut-price stall in the market: like every chef, he knows that his reputation depends on using ingredients of the highest quality. It's the same with herbs. The highest-quality herbs, lovingly produced by organic or biodynamic methods, or carefully harvested in the wild, will work far better than cheaper mass-produced herbs grown with agrochemicals. Buy the best you can afford.

How did it go?

Q   **I've noticed that many of the herbal remedies I see in health-food shops have more than one herb in them. Why is this?**

A   *Good teamwork is common in the herbal world. Herbalists mix and match for two reasons: first, because there are herbs that work particularly well together, in formulae that have been handed down through generations of herbalists. Second, because they want more than one effect: a cough medicine, for instance, might contain herbs that soothe inflamed irritated tissue, antiseptic herbs to help clear infection, herbs to help relax tense constricted bronchi, and herbs to help break up and expel deposits of clogging mucus.*

Q   **I'm completely ignorant about herbal remedies, but I'd love to start experimenting. What would you suggest?**

A   *Begin with my own personal favourite: the orange-flowered marigold, commonly known as calendula (the first part of its Latin name, Calendula officinalis), and a wonderful antiseptic, healing, anti-inflammatory and pain-soothing herb. Dab the lotion on festering newly pierced ears; use it to clean up grazes and cuts; soak an infected finger in an eggcupful of hot water with a splash of tincture in it; treat infected red and swollen sores with a hot compress of lotion, then cover with a dollop of the ointment on a bandage or plaster. Keep a pad of cotton wool soaked in the lotion over an aching infected gum or tooth, apply a squiggle of the ointment on a tissue to relieve swollen, painful piles, and use it to help clear up varicose ulcers or bedsores.*

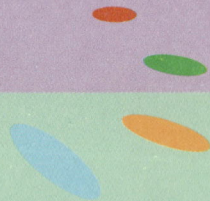

2

Tired all the time

It's normal to feel tired at the end of the day.

But if you feel tired all the time, if you even wake up tired, you're in trouble.

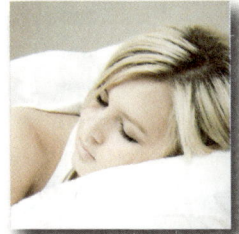

If you suffer from this kind of chronic, day-after-day fatigue, you should check it out with your doctor. There could be good medical reasons for your fatigue – anaemia, diabetes, an under-active thyroid, to name just three – and you need proper treatment for them.

There are some pretty amazing herbs which can help boost your energy, increase your resistance, and raise your spirits, but before you start spending good money on herbal remedies, you need to check out just what's going on to cause your fatigue.

There could be a dozen different causes. You're not eating properly. You're working too hard. You're a born worrier; you can't stop even at bedtime. You're not getting enough exercise. You're bored with your job, or miserable in your love life, or stressed-out by ongoing money anxieties. All or any of these factors can bring on an aching, miserable tiredness that takes all the fun out of living, so study lifestyle factors first and work out what needs fixing.

Here's an idea for you...

If you're burning the midnight oil, if you need to stay sharp and focused for an exam or if you're battling a long demanding job, guarana is the herb for you. This extraordinary tonic from the Amazon rainforest (it's gathered sustainably by local people) can help keep you going cheerfully for hour after hour, with a clear mind, even on minimal sleep – though when the job is done, you'll need to crash out in earnest. Don't drink coffee when you're taking it. Faced with an implacable deadline for delivering a book, I once sailed through three days of intensive work on just four hours' sleep a night and a twice-daily dose of this wonder-working herb. Then I collapsed...

Too much stress can leave you worn out and exhausted. Step forward the great adaptogenic herbs – so-called because they help you 'adapt' to stress by increasing your general resistance and vitality, and so help you cope better with both physical and mental stress. Siberian ginseng is the star in this field, following dozens of studies in the USSR: Russia's athletes and cosmonauts are among its biggest fans. 'An ideal all-round energy tonic,' says UK herbalist Penelope Ody, 'ideal to take whenever extra energy is needed... before a particularly busy period at work, during exams, or before long-distance air travel, for instance.' You can take it for up to six weeks at a time: then you need a fortnight's break. Don't use in an acute infection or if you're on digoxin.

Another great herbal tonic comes from Russian folk medicine. For centuries the roots of *Rhodiola rosea* or Arctic root, were chewed to stave off fatigue and exhaustion, and boost general endurance. Studies carried out by modern Russian researchers have demonstrated this useful property in – among other subjects – sleep-deprived doctors, hard-worked army cadets and students facing key exams.

It sounds blindingly obvious, but lots of people never seem to figure out that their tiredness is caused by a serious sleep shortfall, either because they stay up too late or because they just can't get to sleep. If you're up till the small hours and then need Big Ben to rouse you for a day's work, the cure could be just some regular early nights. If sleep eludes you, even when you retire at a virtuously early hour, try my favourite cure for insomnia – passionflower. I usually take a dose of the tincture an hour or so before bedtime. Valerian, every GP's favourite tranquilliser a century ago, doesn't suit everyone, but when it does, it works brilliantly: it's often combined with sedative hops and wild lettuce. Limeflowers and chamomile – often combined in tea bags or ready-made herbal remedies – both make wonderfully calming bedtime drinks. Sip them slowly while having a bedtime bath to which you've added 10–12 drops of any of the following calming and soothing essential oils: chamomile, lavender or neroli. (Stir the oils into a little whole milk before adding them; they will disperse better.)

'Fatigue makes cowards of us all.'
VINCE LOMBARDI, famous US football coach

Defining idea...

7

How did it go?

Q   **I have a heavy workload, and I often feel run-down, tired and irritable. Can you suggest a really good tonic?**

A   *Try nettles. Yes, those common stinging ones. They're a fantastic pick-me-up because they're loaded with useful minerals, including plenty of iron. In springtime, don rubber gloves to harvest plenty of the tender, fresh young plants, then cook them like spinach, or add to soups or stews. At other times, buy a packet of the dried leaves, brew up a pot of nettle tea – it has a hearty, green taste – and drink it two or three times a day. You can buy nettles in tincture form, too, or in tea bags.*

Q   **I'd like a good pick-me-up for the end of a long day – preferably an alcoholic one. Can you suggest something?**

A   *Try a glass of rosemary wine – very popular with the French, since rosemary is a terrific tonic. To make it, take a good handful of fresh rosemary and strip the leaves off the tough stems. Wash the leaves, dry well, and add them to a bottle of white wine. Seal it again, let it infuse for a week, and take a glassful before supper.*

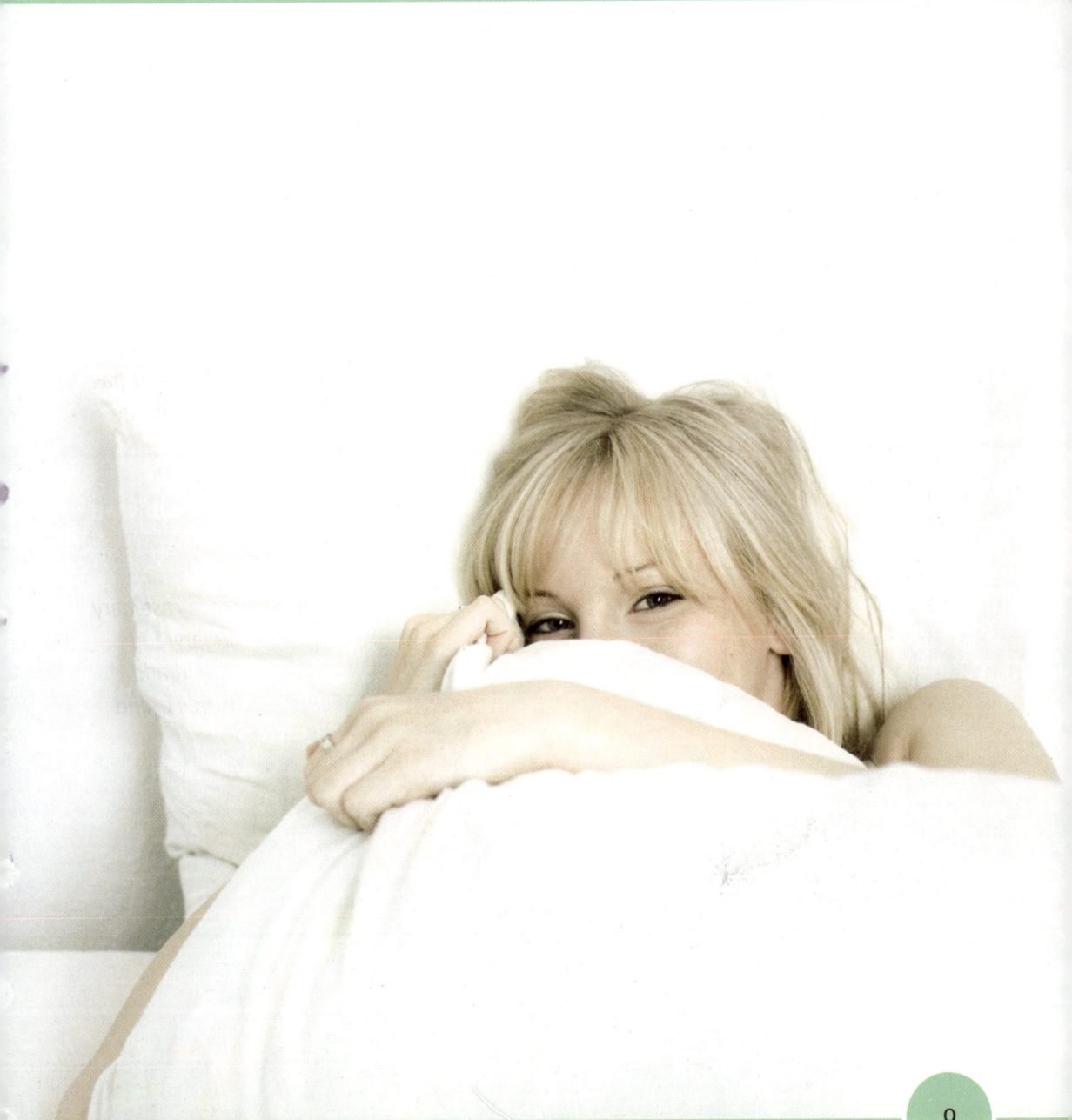

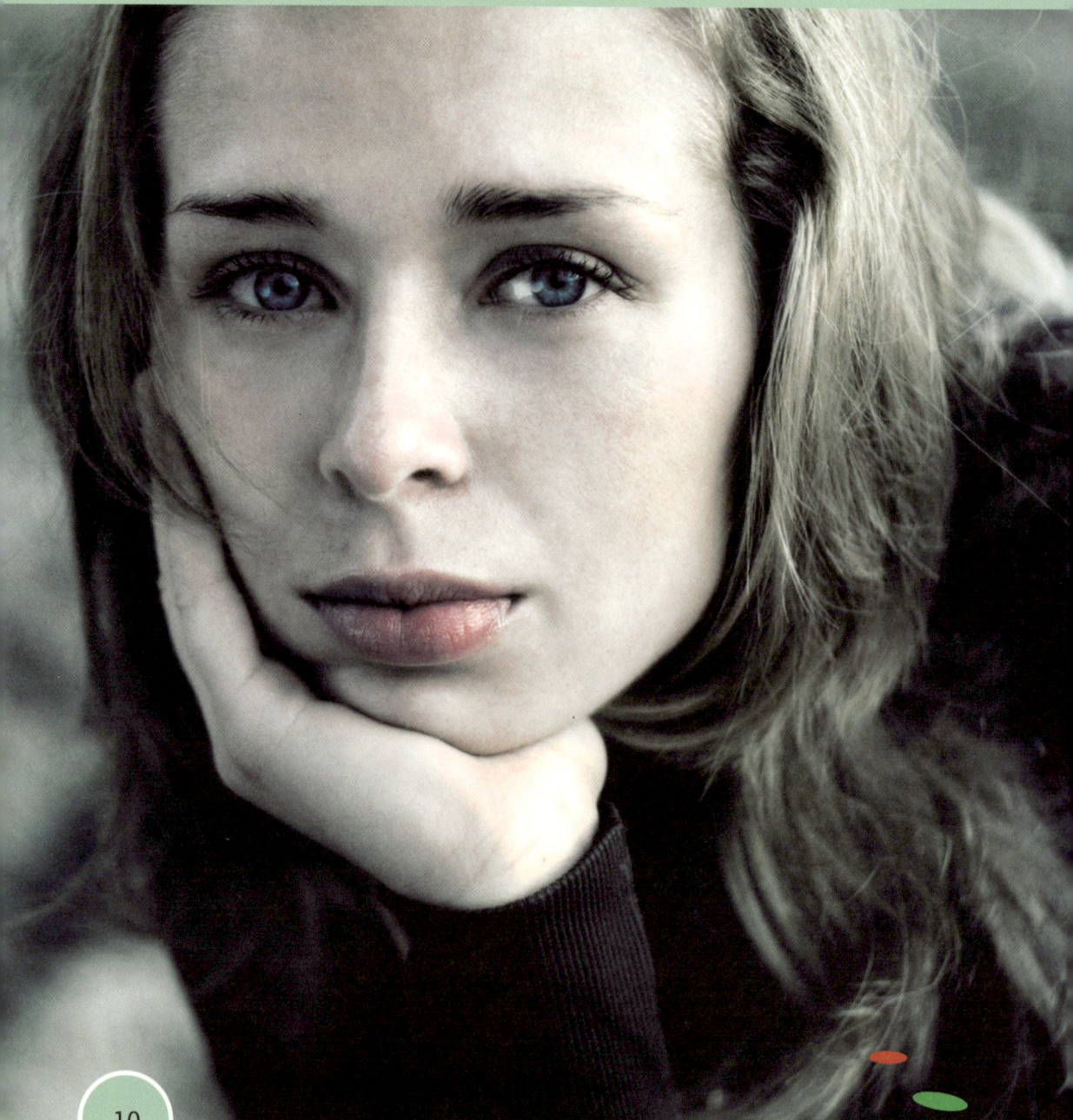

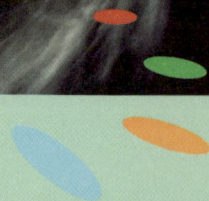

3

The moody blues

If depression is your habitual state of mind, a settled, permanent gloom impossible to snap out of, you need professional advice.

If, though, it comes and goes, hitting just when life is getting you down, there's plenty you can do for yourself. And herbs can lend a great helping hand.

Over long centuries a number of plants have been identified that can help raise the spirits, bring a little light into darkened lives, and soothe the stress and fatigue which tip so many people into depression.

Of course, there's a lot you need to do for yourself before calling on the plants. Believe it or not, diet is a huge contributing factor. Our brains and nervous systems all need good nourishment, not a diet from which the goodness has been processed and refined out. They need the B vitamins: abundant in wheatgerm – there are very few in unfortified white bread – in brown rice and in nuts and seeds, especially almonds, walnuts and sunflower seeds. (If you eat meat, it's also a good source of B vitamins.) And they need the magnesium found in wholegrains, nuts and seeds. Studies have found severe deficiencies of these nutrients in depressed patients.

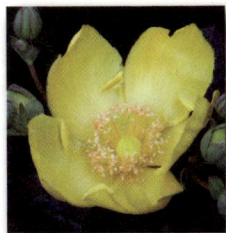

Here's an idea for you...

Buy a pot of lemon balm and keep it on a sunny windowsill. Crush a leaf and smell that warm, uplifting, citrussy fragrance. Lemon balm has a centuries-old reputation as a feel-good mood-lifter for when you're feeling cold, down and miserable: 'powerfully chasing away melancholy', as one seventeenth-century writer put it. Put a small handful of leaves in a mug, fill with boiling water and steep, covered, for ten minutes. Drink this three times a day.

Lack of exercise is certainly another factor, and one recently published study found that exercise was just as effective as prescription drugs in patients with major depressive disorders. Add sunlight and brisk walks in the countryside to your agenda, and your health will improve as well as your mood.

St John's wort blooms at midsummer, producing those gorgeous bright yellow flowers which seem to have sunshine locked into them. For centuries it has been used as folk medicine for the blues, and a huge volume of modern research has turned it into a strong rival for drugs treating minor depression. Unlike drugs such as Prozac and Seroxat, it is generally safe, with few side effects: in one study of 3250 patients taking St John's wort, only 2.5% reported side effects, and those were milder than with conventional drugs. It may be more effective, too. In a German study reported in the *British Medical Journal* in February 2005, 571 patients were treated with the drug paroxetine (Seroxat) or with a standardised extract of St John's wort. Half of those taking the extract reported an improvement, compared to a third taking paroxetine.

Appropriately, this sunshine herb is also effective for SAD patients. Lack of the bright daylight in which humankind evolved is another factor that in itself can tip people into the form of depression aptly known as SAD – seasonal affective disorder – which strikes as the days shorten into winter.

St John's wort needs to be taken for up to six weeks before the effects show up. And don't take it if you are on any prescription medication, including the contraceptive pill, or pregnant or breastfeeding, without consulting either your doctor or a professional herbalist. One added caution: St John's wort can have a very rare side effect – that of sensitising the skin to sunshine. So don't take it if you are having any kind of laser treatment.

'In 1979 a Harvard study showed a majority of those suffering from these conditions (stress, anxiety and depression) preferred alternative and complementary methods over traditional psychotherapy or drugs.'
DR DAVID SERVAN-SCHREIBER,
Healing without Freud or Prozac

Defining idea...

The sunshine herb doesn't work for everyone. If you've tried it without success, a good alternative might be skullcap. It's one of the first plants a herbalist might consider when treating patients whose depression comes chiefly from exhaustion and nervous debility, as well as the post-flu blues which most of us have experienced.

Then there are the great adaptogens. These are a special class of herbs which earn the name because they are non-toxic plants that act to enhance resistance to stress and fatigue, and improve bodily function overall. Siberian ginseng and Arctic (or golden) root are two others. Both have been shown to help depressed patients by boosting general vitality and energy. Siberian ginseng works especially well if you are tired and under constant exhausting pressure. Don't take it, though, if you have an acute infection, and after taking it for six weeks, give yourself a two-week break before starting again. Again, keep your doctor in the picture.

How did it go?

Q **I've heard that omega-3 oils might help my depression. What are they, and where do I find them?**

A *They're a class of essential fatty acids which are critical to the health of every single cell in our bodies. If nerve and brain cells are starved of those vital fatty acids, depression can be one consequence. Oily fish are rich in them. So is linseed oil, made from the seeds of the little blue flax flower. Dozens of studies have shown how vital the omega 3s are as prime treatment for mental and emotional well-being. So eat oily fish, and stock up on linseed oil (also called flaxseed oil) or seeds at your local health food store. Make them a regular part of your daily diet and feel your mood lift. One thing: linseed oil is extremely unstable so buy a reliable brand in a dark bottle, keep it in your fridge and use it up quickly.*

Q **I've heard that some other foods can really help improve depression. Is this so?**

A *Yes, oats. They're a wonderful nerve food, terrific for nervous exhaustion and general debility. Herbalists use a tincture made from the whole oat plant, often combining it with skullcap. There are some excellent products available. Try them – or just eat porridge for breakfast!*

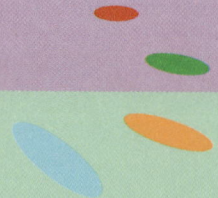

4

Working wonders – when you're wound up like a clockwork toy

Worn out by your high-pressure life? Exhausted by the end of the day? Working till late into the night? Too tired to enjoy the weekend? Too wired to sleep?

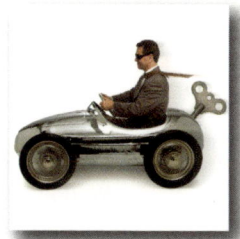

Join the club: stress is the number one ailment of modern Western-style societies.

But don't turn to the classic pick-me-ups of caffeine or alcohol. They may help you get through a rough day but they'll do nothing for your resistance and general health in the long run. Instead, try some great stress-busting herbs, with centuries-old reputations for helping you unwind.

If the stress is ongoing with little sign of any let-up, think adaptogens. That's the name coined in Russia for a small and highly specialised class of medicinal herbs – super-tonics that boost general resistance and help you adapt both physically and mentally to ongoing stress.

The most recently-discovered is Siberian ginseng (*Eleutherococcus senticosus*) which has been researched since the 1950s in Russia. In studies involving thousands of people, it has dramatically improved resistance to extreme working conditions, disease, the

Here's an idea for you...

Trying to cut down on your caffeine intake? Try rooibos or red bush tea from South Africa. It is caffeine free, great for the digestion, rich in minerals and loaded with antioxidants. It has a slightly odd aroma, but a nice round rich taste. Comfortingly, you can drink it with milk like ordinary tea. And while it works as a great pick-me-up during the day, it will help you calm down and sleep well at night-time. What more could you ask of a cuppa?

stress of surgery and the toxic drugs of chemotherapy. Siberian ginseng is usually taken in courses of forty days at a time, with a two- to three-week interval. Side effects are very rare, and usually only at high doses, but can include insomnia and anxiety.

Ashwaganda is a key herb in Ayurveda, the thousands-year-old traditional medicine of India, and since – unlike ginseng – it grows easily and happily from seed around the world, it has become increasingly popular with Western herbalists faced with deeply stressed patients. 'An exceptional nerve tonic – one of the best remedies for stress,' says UK herbalist Anne McIntyre, who has big healthy green plants of it growing in her Cotswold herb garden. 'From my observation of patients taking ashwaganda over a period of four to six weeks, it certainly helps to enhance energy and positivity, engender calmness and clarity, improve memory and concentration, and promote restful sleep.'

Rhodiola, a little plant grown in the Arctic mountains of Siberia, is a relative newcomer to Western herbalists, but it has already made a name for itself as a great tonic for people in demanding, high-pressure jobs. When you're tired, depressed and low in energy, rhodiola might be the one for you. It's been little studied in the West, but Russian researchers tested it successfully in exhausted young doctors working impossible hours and stressed students facing exams, among other subjects.

With any of these adaptogens, look for a reliable brand, and follow the manufacturer's dosage suggestions.

'*You don't get ulcers from what you eat. You get ulcers from what's eating you.* '
VICKI BAUM, American writer

Defining idea...

There are numbers of other herbs with a reputation for effective stress-busting: among them limeflowers, skullcap, hops, passionflower, lemon balm, valerian and oats. Any health-food shop will offer a range of tablets, tinctures or teas featuring these lifesavers in various combinations. Here's a rundown of what they – and others – can do to help you calm down and sort yourself out when things are really getting to you.

Herbalists prescribe oats – usually in the form of a tincture of both grains and the grassy bits – for nervous prostration, exhaustion, depression: wonderfully nourishing for the nervous system. It is often combined with passionflower which is wonderful for insomnia, easing you into restful sleep.

Skullcap is one of the most widely used nerve tonics, almost specific for severe nervous tension. Limeflowers help relax you when you feel strung up, soothing those nervous jitters. And lemon balm is another great remedy for nervous tension, especially the kind that gets to your guts.

Prisoners, like commuters, are powerless people, but in one south London jail, according to a *Times* report early in 2004, the staff were dishing out herbal teas instead of sedatives in the evening – to the enthusiastic approval of the inmates, particularly the women. The two chosen varieties of tea, formulated by herbalist Dr Malcolm Stuart, contained top stress-busting herbs such as limeflowers, hops, passionflower, valerian root and skullcap, together with gut-calming fennel and yarrow, and sedative hawthorn.

How did it go?

Q I have important exams coming up, I'll need to burn the midnight oil, putting in extra study, and I can't take those gallons of coffee. Is there any herbal alternative I could use?

A *Go for guarana, an amazing herb from the Brazilian Amazon, which is popular with long-haul aircrews. It contains some caffeine – a daily dose has less than one cup of tea – but other ingredients slow down and cushion its impact. Guarana helps you to stay hard at work, feeling clear-minded and cheerful, on minimal sleep for two to three days at a time, but then you'll really need a break and a good rest.*

Q I often work late, come home and fall into bed – then I can't sleep. Can you help?

A *Try a hot lavender footbath. Add 5 drops of the essential oil to a little milk, tip it into a hot footbath, and soak your feet in this for five to ten minutes while you sip a calming chamomile tea. Put a drop of lavender oil on your pillow, too.*

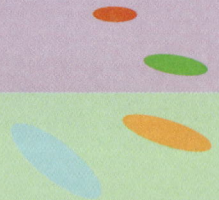

5

The aching brow

Everybody has experienced a headache at one time or another in their lives.

Indigestion, eyestrain, tiredness, stress, liver upsets, menstrual problems, high blood pressure can all bring on that horrid throbbing pain…

If you only get a headache now and then, you'll probably swallow a painkiller and be done with it. But if you're a regular victim or a migraine sufferer, herbal medicine has a lot to offer.

Tension headaches are the commonest kind. They're caused by tightened muscles in the neck and shoulders – just where most people store their stress – or in the scalp. Its easy to work out if your headache is this kind: just soak a cloth in scalding hot water and apply it to the aching area. If this feels comforting, try soaking the cloth in a hot tea made by steeping 5–6 sprigs of fresh rosemary in a big mug of boiling water, covered, for ten minutes. Then strain the liquid and drink half; use the rest for your compress. Internally, rosemary helps dilate constricted blood vessels, and it's a great general pick-me-up.

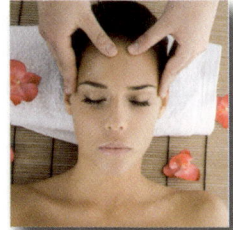

Here's an idea for you...

Some headaches are caused by painful constriction of blood vessels in the back of the neck. Try applying a hot wheatbag or hot water bottle. Interestingly, if this brings some relief, a dose of feverfew will also help.

Over-dilated blood vessels can produce that horrid throbbing pain too, usually around the temples and forehead. Try cooling either chamomile or limeflower tea (use a tea bag) right down until it's ice cold. Then use it on a compress to calm down those blood vessels.

An unhappy gut often brings on that throbbing head. If this is your problem, herbalist David Hoffmann suggests a trio of helpful herbs. Make a tea with equal parts of meadowsweet – the plant from which aspirin was originally derived – and calming lemon balm and lavender. Or a nice cup of refreshing peppermint tea might just do the trick, especially if you have the tea bags at hand.

There's nothing new about migraine, so it's not surprising that the two most popular herbal remedies for it have been used in folk medicine for centuries. One is feverfew: an eighteenth-century English doctor wrote of one lady he knew 'that having in the younger part of her life a very terrible and almost constant Headache, fixed in one small spot, and raging at all times almost to distraction, she was at length cured by a maidservant with this herb'. Like many brilliant herbal remedies, feverfew was forgotten – until trials at the London Migraine Clinic in the 1980s gave impressive results, and other research carried out since has confirmed their findings. Feverfew seems to work for about two in three sufferers and it works best when it's taken fresh – a lot of its fans simply grow this attractive plant and eat a few (one to four) of the fresh leaves a day in a sandwich. However, they taste off-puttingly bitter and they can give you nasty little mouth ulcers and a sore tongue, so you might prefer the tablet or tincture form of the freeze-dried fresh leaves, taken first thing in the morning. You need to take it regularly as a preventive, and pregnant or breastfeeding women should avoid it.

The other great – and recently rediscovered – migraine herb is the root of butterbur (*Petasites hybridus*), an attractive wild flower with dense cones of pink and white flowers. There has only been limited testing of this plant for safety and efficacy. However, in a recent clinical trial carried out in the US, and published in the journal *Neurology*, 68% of patients taking two 75mg tablets daily of a proprietary preparation experienced a drop of at least 50% in the frequency and severity of their migraines. Butterbur contains some dodgy chemicals called pyrrolizidine alkaloids, now linked with damage to the liver. Look for brands from which these 'PA's have been removed. And – as with all medicines – don't take them if you are pregnant.

Herbalists use valerian as a general calmer and muscle-relaxant, useful for anxiety or sleeplessness, as well as for the terrible tensed muscles of chronic stress. But unlike conventional tranquillisers, it will help you relax both physically and mentally without blurring your 'edge' or making you feel drowsy. To enhance its effect, it's sometimes combined with lemon balm, a wonderful herb for calming frazzled nerves and untying tension knots.

If valerian doesn't work for you – and if you're suffering from depression, don't even try it – another great muscle-relaxant is skullcap, which works particularly well with feverfew.

'For some people, a migraine is literally the only thing that can get them to rest – in silence, in a dark room. It is an anguished effort by the body to get the rest it needs.'
UK herbalist MICHAEL MCINTYRE

Defining idea...

How did it go?

Q **I've heard that peppermint can help a headache. How would you take it?**

A *Steep a few sprigs of peppermint in boiling water, covered, for five minutes, then drink most of it. Cool the rest, soak a cloth in it, and use it as a compress on your forehead or the back of your neck, wherever the pain is worst. You can also find roller balls with helpful essential oils to apply to forehead and neck: look for peppermint, rosemary or chamomile.*

Q **Someone told me that ginger was good for migraines. Is this correct?**

A *There's no hard evidence, but some Danish researchers reckoned that since ginger has a high reputation for neurological problems in the traditional medicine of India, it might work. So they suggested powdered ginger to a woman who had had severe migraines for sixteen years. Take it, they suggested, at the first sign of one. It stopped her migraines so successfully that she began eating a daily dose. I passed on this tip to a colleague who suffered regular agonising migraines. She found that if she took a big dose of ginger (in capsule form) at the very first sign of a migraine, it simply stopped. The dose that worked for her was 500–600mg of powdered ginger in capsules. Worth a try?*

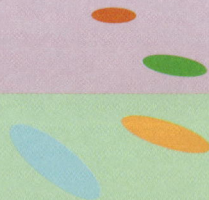

6

Losing the plot

Always losing your glasses? Can't remember the names of your friends' children? Forget what you went to your bedroom to pick up? Worried you're getting senile?

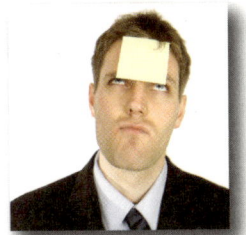

Some of the most exciting herbal research over the last few decades has shown that certain herbs can work to boost memory and general alertness.

Top of the list, and a global bestseller, is an extract from the leaves of *Ginkgo biloba*, the oldest living tree: it's been around for an estimated 200 million years and individual trees can live up to 1000 years. Appropriately, this grand survivor is turning out to be the best-ever friend of the elderly. Twentieth-century research in Germany revealed its power to increase blood flow in the brain and thus help boost memory, concentration and mental performance. So impressive are its powers that in just one year – 1988 – German doctors wrote over five million prescriptions for it. It doesn't just help improve memory: it can also help reduce the absent-mindedness, anxiety and confusion so often experienced by elderly people along with that fading recall.

Here's an idea for you...

If you face of hours of taxing mental desk work, put some rosemary essential oil in a burner next to your desk. It will help keep you calm as well as alert.

It also appears to delay the onset of full-blown dementia. In 2002, the UK's Alzheimer's Society published the biggest ever comprehensive review on the use of ginkgo for the treatment of dementia, examining thirty-three previous clinical trials dating back to 1976. The new research, they concluded, provided promising evidence that taking ginkgo can improve memory and overall function for people with dementia.

But it's not just the elderly who can profit from its memory-boosting powers: herbal students have been known to dose up on it before exams, and claim they feel sharper, more alert. In a small study, participants given a single quite large dose of ginkgo found their general alertness and speed of reaction had sharpened quite noticeably two and a half hours later – an effect still noticeable six hours afterwards.

Most people seem able to take ginkgo, even over long periods of time, without serious side effects. But if you are taking aspirin, blood-thinning drugs, anticonvulsants or antidepressants, consult your doctor or a medical herbalist. And don't take it if you are pregnant or breastfeeding.

Three other herbs – all from the Far East – that work to boost memory and concentration are gotu kola from India, ginseng from China and Korea, and Siberian ginseng. They're often combined with ginkgo to even greater effect. Gotu kola, a little creeping waterside plant, was the favourite forage plant of the Ceylon elephants, incidentally – whose long memories are proverbial. Good ginseng is expensive but Siberian Ginseng is much less so, and in trials on workers carrying out mental tasks such as proofreading, it gave them a distinct edge over those taking a dummy pill. Don't take it if you have an acute infection.

Defining idea…

'God gave us memories that we might have roses in December.'
J. M. BARRIE, *Courage*

But the Far East certainly doesn't have a monopoly of plants that boost your brainpower and memory. 'There's rosemary, that's for remembrance,' says Shakespeare's Ophelia to Hamlet. Modern research has pinpointed two reasons why rosemary deserves its age-old reputation. First, it helps preserve levels of a brain chemical called acetylcholine, a key worker in the area of the brain where memories are created and stored: it transports information between brain cells. If your acetylcholine levels are inadequate, or the chemical is broken down too quickly, then you too could start to become dozy, forgetful and absentminded. Low levels in the brain are a key indication of Alzheimer's. Almost all the famous plant boosters of brain function – and most of the new drugs – work to conserve this chemical, so regular doses of rosemary could help sharpen you up amazingly.

How should you take rosemary? Well, have an early morning cuppa of rosemary tea: infuse 3–4 young top shoots in a cup of boiling water, covered, for five minutes, then strain and drink. This pale green brew is wonderfully invigorating. And if you have a pick-me-up morning bath, add 10 drops of rosemary essential oil in a cup of whole milk under the running tap. Even the aroma of this plant is enlivening. Interestingly, the young flowering tops of rosemary and sage are much richer in antioxidants than the older, woodier leaves and stalks further down. Plants are like people; our ability to make and store antioxidants declines with age.

Sage, wrote a sixteenth-century English herbalist, 'is singularly good for the head and quickeneth the nerves and memory'. For centuries this observation was written off as just the sort of rubbish you'd expect to find in quaint old herbals. But researchers at the Universities of Northumbria and Newcastle recently took another look at sage, and found that it did indeed improve memory: in a small clinical trial with healthy, young adults, those who had taken sage performed significantly better in a word recall test.

How did it go?

Q   I have important exams coming up and I'd love something to take to help me sharpen up my wits. Any suggestions?

A   *Herbalist Jill Davies suggests prickly ash, a wonderful wake-up herb. 'It will assist', she says, 'where the brain in particular feels foggy and slow, quickly bringing clarity and a feeling of uplift and energy'. Try it in tincture form. Or take a daily dose of ginkgo – I know at least three herbalists who take a morning shot of ginkgo on days when they're going to need all their wits about them.*

Q   I'm in my fifties and I'm anxious to keep my memory functioning well, but I don't want to swallow more pills. Is there a pleasant herb tea you could suggest?

A   *Try lemon balm, which will flourish in your garden or in a window box. Infuse 15–20 of the fresh leaves in a cupful of boiling water for five minutes, covered, then strain and drink. It's another herb with a long reputation as an aid to memory. The seventeenth-century diarist John Evelyn was quoting contemporary doctors when he wrote that 'Balm is sovereign for the brain, strengthening the memory and powerfully chasing away melancholy'.*

7

Saturday night fever

**Everybody remembers the worst hangover they ever had...
the nausea, giddiness, crushing headache, distraught
stomach and total physical prostration.**

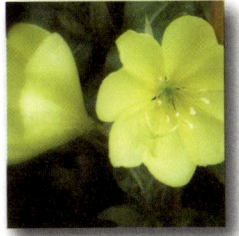

Few hangovers are as bad as this,
fortunately, but if you suffer the occasional lesser
hangover, it's good to know of a few herbal
tricks for damage limitation.

Hangovers produce a wide range of disagreeable sensations. Nausea? Damage to
your stomach lining inflicted by the alcohol and its by-products inside your
digestive system. Headache, dry mouth and general shakiness? That's dehydration,
as your kidneys work overtime to offload all that toxic garbage. Physical prostration?
It's down to severe malnutrition, since all that booze has seriously depleted levels of
essential nutrients.

High up on this list are essential fatty acids, and the oil extracted from the beautiful
yellow-flowered evening primrose comes to the rescue here. Its yield of one key
essential fatty acid was demonstrated in the early 80s, and a bunch of Harvard
medical students figured that this might make the stuff good news for a hangover.

Here's an idea for you...

In my occasionally misspent youth, I once came across a herbal tea which actually helped soothe a hangover quite quickly. It was formulated, I discovered, by herbalist Jill Davies, and it was made with equal parts of limeflower, spearmint, rosemary leaf, lemon balm, lavender flowers and a dash of peppermint oil – a wonderful mix of calming, cheering and reviving herbs, with the peppermint oil doing wonders to soothe your tormented gut. If you don't have the original blend to hand, an infusion of limeflower or rosemary or lavender to which you add 2–3 drops of peppermint oil will still help.

In an informal little trial they all swallowed half a dozen 500mg capsules of the oil after a heavy evening, and reported that they didn't feel nearly as bad as they deserved to next morning. Better still, take a couple of capsules before you start the evening, and another two before you go to bed – if you remember.

By the way, gin, vodka and white wine may not contain less alcohol than dark rum, sherry, bourbon whisky, brandy, port and red wine, but they're less loaded with substances called congeners, toxic by-products of the fermentation process. In one study, 33% of those who drank an amount of bourbon relative to their body weight reported a severe hangover, compared to only 3% of those who drank the same amount of vodka.

Your liver works overtime when you're hung over, struggling to metabolise all that alcohol and help clear it from your system. Milk thistle is one herb all regular drinkers should get to know if they value the health of their poor long-suffering livers. Its seeds exert a protective and regenerative effect on the liver, stimulating the production of enzymes which help speed recovery from that hangover and general detoxification. Another wonderful tonic for the liver is the bitter-tasting root of the common dandelion, which not only stimulates liver function but supplies minerals depleted by boozing.

Herbs with a specially bitter taste are the drinker's friend, because they help the liver cope with the digestive havoc that goes with a hangover. This is why so many of these herbs have been used to create the post-dinner drinks the French call 'digestifs' – and why they can work as hangover cures.

'I feel sorry for people who don't drink. When they wake up in the morning, that's as good as they're going to feel all day long.'
DEAN MARTIN

Defining
idea...

Absinthe, made from bitter wormwood, and up to 95° proof, was long popular in Paris's Left Bank. Fernet Branca, made from forty different herbs and spices macerated for a year in pure alcohol, tastes so vilely bitter that you couldn't possibly drink it unless you were badly hung over. (I still remember marvelling during one holiday at a friend of mine who used to stagger to the beach bar in Marbella every morning, and order a large Fernet Branca on the rocks for breakfast.)

Angostura Bitters, confusingly, are *not* made from the bark of the Angostura tree, medicinal though it is, but from another famously bitter herb, gentian, together with some gut-soothing spices. (The Bitters were so-called because they were devised by a German doctor based in Angostura, Venezuela, for his dyspeptic patients.) The British naval favourite of pink gin is made healthier for livers by the dash of Angostura Bitters it contains, and US herbal expert James Duke suggests making an anti-hangover drink by adding a few drops of Bitters to a glass of hot water.

Don't ask me why, but tomatoes are a known hangover remedy: they're rich in vitamin C and wonder-working compounds called flavonoids. Hot chilli peppers are an unrivalled pick-me-up and most traditional hangover remedies contain a shot of hot cayenne. Try stirring a good dash of cayenne into a glass of tomato juice.

How did it go?

Q   I feel really sick to my stomach when I'm hung over. Is there any herb you can suggest?

A   Certainly: try ginger. It's fabulous for any kind of sickness, including seasickness. If you have fresh root ginger to hand, grate a plump inch of it into a mug, fill it with boiling water and let the ginger steep, covered, for ten minutes. Then strain and drink. Dried ginger works well too: stir half a teaspoonful into warm water with honey.

Q   I don't suppose there's a herb that would make me drink less, is there?

A   Actually there is. It's a herb called kudzu from the Far East, which is the chief component of an ancient Chinese formula popularly known as the 'drunkenness dispeller' because of its ability to inhibit the craving for alcohol, slow consumption, and diminish the morning-after effects. In a recent double-blind trial at a US hospital researchers found that moderately heavy drinkers, given a kudzu extract in capsule form for a week before taking part in a drinking experiment, consumed significantly less alcohol than those given dummy pills. All the subjects except one reduced their intake. On average, alcohol consumption was cut by almost 50% and researchers also noted that subjects drank more slowly, taking longer to finish each beer.

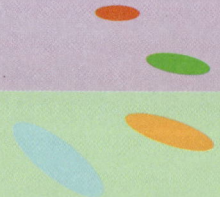

8
Counting sheep

Find yourself dreading bedtime and the long sleepless night ahead?

Try one of the numbers of tried-and-trusted herbal remedies to help you nod off tonight.

Stress, anxiety, depression, late nights, jangled nerves, a blazing row with a loved one, a strong after-dinner espresso, long sessions staring into your computer screen or too much late-night TV – any of these can mess up your sleep for the night, leaving you tossing and turning, dozing fitfully and waking in the morning feeling like a rag. Prescription sleeping pills aren't the best answer: they may knock you out, but they reduce the amount of quality sleep you get and can leave you feeling frowsty and hungover the next day. There's a danger of addiction, too, if you become dependent on them.

Herbs aren't addictive in this chemical sense, although if you get to rely on them, they could become psychological crutches instead. The sleep they encourage is a sound healthy snooze: you'll wake fresh and alert, and you don't even need a prescription for them.

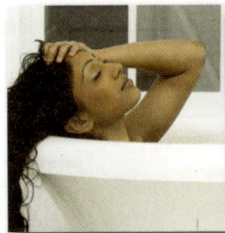

Here's an idea for you... **Try a comforting bedtime bath. Add 10–15 drops of good essential oil – such as lavender, orange blossom (aka neroli) or the sweet and exotic ylang-ylang – to the bath water. These aren't just great smells: they are absorbed into the bloodstream through the skin in a matter of minutes to travel the body and work their calming, soothing effect where needed. Relax in this lovely bath for twenty minutes then go straight to bed. Be careful not to apply these oils undiluted to your skin: a good way to disperse them through the bath water is to add them to a cupful of whole milk first and pour them in together.**

If you grow herbs, you may already have lemon balm in your garden. This attractive bright green herb with its lovely lemony smell is a famed cheerer of the spirits: it also calms the digestive system, relaxes strung-up nerves and encourages soothing sleep. It is especially good for those kept awake by stress or depression. Pick a good tablespoonful of the fresh leaves, put them in a mug, fill it with boiling water and let it steep, covered, for a few minutes before straining it and drinking at bedtime. Drink it during the day, too, instead of tea or coffee. The sedative and gut-calming effects of lemon balm, incidentally, are recognised by Commission E, for years the official German advisory body on herb safety and efficacy.

Another great herb for the sleeplessness brought on by stress or anxiety is valerian, which will help you feel sleepy if you take it at bedtime – you can take it during the day, too, to help cope with stress. In one clinical study, 89% of the subjects reported improved sleep, and 44% 'perfect sleep'. The remaining 11% probably included some of the small number of people for whom valerian not only doesn't work, but can leave feeling wired up instead. As a sleep aid, valerian is often combined with lemon balm or hops.

People have been known to fall asleep in hop warehouses, and many people swear by a hop pillow to help them nod off. It's the relaxing aroma of the essential oils in those little papery cones which will keep you sleeping soundly all night. Lots of ready-made herbal remedies for sleeplessness contain hops, or you can order a supply and make up your own tea: infuse a teaspoonful of the dried heads in a cupful of boiling water, covered, for a few minutes, and drink at bedtime. There's a caveat about hops: if it's depression that's wrecking your slumbers, avoid them – they might make it worse. The same applies to valerian.

'In the real dark night of the soul, it is always three o'clock in the morning.'
F. SCOTT FITZGERALD

Defining idea...

Chamomile is another great stress-busting herb; drink it during the day as well as at bedtime. Note that the average chamomile tea bag contains a dose herbalists would consider laughably small, so order it in loose form and use a tablespoonful to a cup of boiling water. Infuse it, covered, for ten minutes.

The famous French herbalist Maurice Messegue once treated a wealthy American woman for chronic insomnia. She had tried everything, she told him. Messegue advised her to eat three lettuces for dinner every night. That Christmas she sent him a greetings card with the words 'I sleep... I sleep...' In fact lettuces contain a milky latex with a known soporific effect, so try making lettuce soup for dinner.

My personal favourite – and many herbalists would agree with me – is passionflower. It's the medicinal kind you want, though, not the ornamental garden flower. I've always found it one of the most effective of gentle sleep inducers. I take a dose of the tincture in a little water half an hour before bedtime, and it rarely fails me.

How did it go?

Q **I've heard that lime leaves can help you sleep and there's a big lime tree in the garden. How do I make it work for me?**

A *Put a generous handful of the leaves or flowers (you can also buy these dried) into a litre of boiling water and simmer, covered, for twenty minutes. Strain and add it to a nice warm bedtime bath. Messegue recalls being put in a lime bath by his father when he was three years old and could not sleep: 'I would actually start to doze off while still in the water.'*

Q **I've tried drinking a herbal cuppa or swallowing various herbal pills at bedtime, but they don't seem to work for me. I have a bath every morning, so I don't want another one at night. Is there anything else I could try?**

A *Go for a hot aromatic footbath instead: the soles of your feet are specially good at absorbing essential oils and experiments have shown that warm feet will help you get to sleep, anyway. Add 2–3 drops of lavender, neroli or chamomile essential oil to a deep bowl of hot water and soak your feet for ten minutes. Then dry them, pull on warm socks and go straight to bed.*

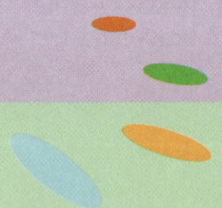

9

Quit your bellyaching

Suffering from indigestion, gas, heartburn and 'acidity'?

Don't go on popping antacids — use kitchen medicine to sort out the problems that start right there.

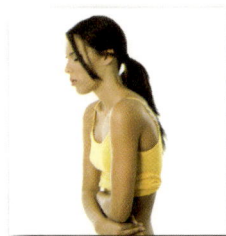

It's not just what you eat but when and how that could be causing your digestive hassle. Too much rich food and drink, smoking, irregular meals, bolting your food down without chewing it properly, grabbing a lunchtime sandwich at your desk, eating when you're extra-stressed, or miserable or in a rage: any of these can give you an unhappy gut. Swallowing an antacid pill may give you instant relief – as those TV commercials invitingly suggest – but it could be a costly habit; your stomach needs acids to digest your lunch, so it will simply step up production, paving the way for tomorrow's gastric ulcer.

A windowsill of fresh herbs in pots and a well-stocked spice rack can do more for your digestive health and happiness than a truckload of antacid pills. Herbs and spices aren't just upmarket flavour enhancers: for thousands of years people all over the planet have been using them as friends to their digestion too. The mints are soothers for the entire gut, effective against gas, cramps, colicky pains. Garlic and onions help you digest rich fatty foods. The cayenne so widely used in hot countries like India and Mexico is powerfully antiseptic, as well as a terrific tonic. Sage, too, is antiseptic, and is traditionally paired with pork to protect against bugs and parasites; it also aids the digestion of rich, heavy food. Caraway seeds or bay leaves can take the wind out of beans and cabbage.

Here's an idea for you...

Nauseous? Try some ginger tea. Grate an inch of fresh root into a mug and cover it with boiling water. Leave it to infuse for five minutes before drinking. Ginger capsules, candied ginger, even ginger ale can work too – but make sure the latter is good quality and actually contains ginger and not just flavourings. Or you could go for ginger teabags.

The warming spices that feature in rich festive fare – cinnamon, cloves, ginger – all boost circulation to aid digestion, and dispel gas from the stomach and intestines. Coriander, beloved in the Middle East, is a cooling spice and another friend to the digestion, while cumin, with its deep sweet pungent flavour, is another favourite anti-wind spice. In the Far East a dash of ginger is added to almost every fish or meat dish to counter toxicity, fire up the taste buds and boost digestion.

And while ulcer-sufferers are usually warned off spicy food, a number of spices have actually been shown to be strongly active against the bug *Helicobacter pylori* now thought to be responsible for stomach ulcers. Among them are turmeric, chilli, caraway and cumin.

Executive stress, excess coffee and alcohol intake, bad eating habits and a wide range of drugs including – yes – aspirin, as well as the non-steroidal anti-inflammatory drugs or NSAIDs swallowed in heroic quantities by arthritis patients, can all help trigger a painful ulcer in the sensitive mucous lining of the gut. The acids our stomachs produce for digestion then burn and irritate the ulcer. A number of herbs can help see off this painful problem: consult a professional herbalist who will help sort it out for you. Among the herbs they're likely to include in a prescription is liquorice, wonderful for acid situations. It foams in the gut and puts a protective layer on the stomach, allowing healing to take place from underneath. Another is slippery elm; it is spectacularly high in mucilage, which once swallowed swells to provide a soft protective coating for the damaged gut lining, soothing inflammation into the bargain.

Linseeds are another wonderful soother for the unhappy and inflamed gut; crush a dessertspoonful of the seeds and drink with a big glass of water. Down in your gut they will swell to soothing jelly that will help calm and heal a troubled gut. Take this half an hour before a meal.

Our modern Western diet is predominantly sweet, salty or bland in taste: what's missing are foods with a bitter taste which stimulate the entire digestive process, all the way down the gut. Selective breeding over centuries has eliminated most of that useful bitterness from our vegetables, though it's still found in some of them – kale, endive and watercress, for example. Herbalists turn to a number of plants with a notably bitter taste to help get gastric juices flowing again and boost production of digestive enzymes. Famous European aperitifs, drunk before meals to sharpen the appetite and improve digestion, are based on bitter-tasting herbs such as gentian and artichoke. Another useful one is centaury: if your whole digestive system is weak and troubled, take 20 drops of the bitter-tasting tincture in a glass of water before meals, twice a day. And when your digestion is complaining after a particularly rich and heavy meal, take a teaspoon of wonderful Swedish Bitters, composed of bitter herbs including gentian, artichoke leaf, centaury, dandelion, blessed thistle and wormwood, balanced by warming aromatic herbs such as fennel, ginger and cardamom. Sorry, you can't get it in pill form: that bitter taste is the whole point. (Don't take it, though, if you're pregnant or breast-feeding, or if you have serious digestive problems.)

The aspirin we all swear by was originally derived from the pretty wild flower meadowsweet. But unlike aspirin, which can actually cause gastric ulcers if overused, the mix of chemicals in meadowsweet work to protect and heal the mucous lining of the stomach. When herbalist Dee Atkinson's father was forbidden tea and coffee because of his painful gastric ulcer, Dee blended a special tea for him starring this helpful herb.

'Each one of the substances of a man's diet acts upon his body and changes it in some way, and upon these changes his whole life depends, whether he be in health, in sickness, or convalescent.'
HIPPOCRATES

Defining idea...

37

How did it go?

Q   **I get a lot of gas and colic after meals. Can you help at all?**

A   *Probably; try this. Crush 25g of caraway seeds, add a cupful of boiling water and infuse them, covered, for twenty minutes (or you can soak the seeds in cold water overnight). Take doses of a couples of tablespoons at intervals until the pain is gone. Caraway seeds are a noted anti-flatulence remedy: in north-European cookery they are often added to windy dishes like cabbage.*

Q   **Indigestion is a real pain for me occasionally. Any suggestions?**

A   *Herbalist Anne McIntyre suggests this calming tisane which will relax tension in the stomach muscles and soothe inflammation in the gut: take 2 teaspoons each of dried chamomile flowers, dried spearmint leaves and dried meadowsweet. Put them in a teapot or jug and pour 600ml of boiling water over them. Infuse for ten to fifteen minutes, and drink a cupful three times a day after meals. If you work away from home take some with you in a little thermos flask.*

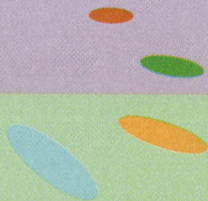

10

Irritable bowel syndrome

Millions of people in the Western world suffer from irritable bowel syndrome: according to some estimates, as many as one in five of us.

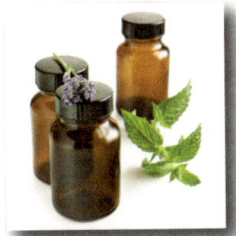

Why? It's down to the dreadful diet that too many of us eat.

Irritable bowel syndrome (IBS) is uncomfortable at best; at worst, it makes life impossible for its victims. The wretched list of symptoms includes cramping pains, gas, bloating, bunged-up constipation or diarrhoea so bad you can't plan an outing without an anxious toilet check. Your doctor may prescribe drugs to relieve these symptoms. But they won't sort out your problems long term. What you need is good old kitchen medicine. And some tried and trusted herbs.

Sensitivity to certain foods is a common cause of IBS. Herbalist Sue Eldin is one of the team at a London medical practice, and about half the cases referred to her by her doctor colleagues are gut disorders. At the first consultation, Sue gives patients a diet diary to be filled in carefully for a fortnight. On one page, the patient notes every single thing eaten or drunk over the course of a day and the time it was taken; on the opposite page, every change in symptoms – and the time the change occurred.

Here's an idea for you...

Horrible griping pains? Try fennel tea. It's so mild that Italian mammas give it to their colicky babies, but it's highly effective for griping pains and wind, especially drunk just after a meal. You can get it as tea bags, or you can try this wonderfully warming brew suggested by the nineteenth-century German herbalist, Abbe Kneipp: 'A spoonful of fennel seed cooked in a cup of milk for five to ten minutes... and drunk as hot as possible.'

At the next consultation, Sue goes through the diary. 'You can often spot the problem straight away,' she says. 'Saccharin is a massive trigger – those dreadful diet foods. So are artificial flavourings and colourings. Monosodium glutamate is one of the worst, omnipresent in our Western diet – packet soups, burgers, crisps. Pork – bacon, salami, pate, sausages and pies. In my experience, though, wheat and dairy products are seldom the problem.'

Once trigger foods are avoided, Sue finds problems often clear up fast. Only then does she prescribe herbs to deal with the distressing symptoms IBS brings in its wake.

Slippery elm is the herb she's most likely to prescribe – one of the most useful herbs English colonists learned about from North American Indians. The inner bark of the elm tree is loaded with mucilage, a smooth slippery substance that coats the walls of the intestines to soothe, protect and heal them. It's nourishing too, and will help clear up diarrhoea. Buy it in pill form or as a powder, and prepare it according to the maker's directions.

The leaves, the flowers and especially the root of marshmallows, closely related to hollyhocks, are also rich in mucilage. Try a tea made from the dried herb: 30g to a litre of boiling water, infused covered for ten minutes, and drunk over the course of the day. Or add 30g of the powdered root to a litre of tepid water, leave for two hours, then very gently warm to just above body temperature. Add a little honey to this wonderfully soothing goo.

'Herb medicine is uniquely suited for the treatment of illness of the digestive system. Throughout the natural world food is medicine, and the same concept applies to herbs – the ultimate medicinal food.'
DAVID HOFFMANN, from *Healthy Digestion*

Defining idea...

'Meadowsweet,' says US herbalist David Hoffmann, 'is one of the best digestive remedies available... it protects and soothes the mucous membranes of the digestive tract, reducing acidity and easing nausea.' Make a tea from this pretty wild flower with its clouds of fragrant creamy blossoms: pour a cupful of boiling water over 2 teaspoons of the dried herb, let it steep for ten to fifteen minutes then drink hot three times a day. You can take it in pill or tincture form, too.

IBS used to be known as spastic colon, from the horrid griping pains it produced as the colon went into spasm. It's peppermint to the rescue here: it works by relaxing those hyperactive muscles in the colon walls, and it helps if you're nauseated too. Peppermint oil is especially popular with IBS sufferers, and in tea form peppermint is so popular that many restaurants will offer it to you instead of an after-dinner coffee.

How did it go?

Q I'm an IBS patient, and the worst of it seems to be severe constipation, which leaves me feeling tired, bloated and miserable. My doctor told me to eat a lot of bran as I need a lot of fibre but, although it helps with the constipation, it seems to make my stomach pains even worse. Is there an alternative?

A *'You may as well eat sawdust,' is Sue Eldin's view of bran. 'It can seriously irritate a sensitive gut.' Instead, go for gentler forms of fibre from fruit and vegetables: raw or stewed apples are one of the best. And try golden linseed which will swell in your intestines to bulk and soften your stools, and trigger peristaltic movement in the gut walls. It also helps soothe and heal the inflamed gut lining. Crush a tablespoonful of the dry seeds and swallow it down with a big glass of water. The water is vital, or the seeds might simply pile up and block your gut. Do this two to three times a day.*

Q I'm told I shouldn't drink too much tea or coffee until my IBS is better. Are there any herbal teas which actually taste nice and will do me a bit of good?

A *Chamomile and peppermint are both first-rate for any digestive problem, but you can get a bit bored with them. Try lemon balm, fresh if possible; otherwise dried. Put a large handful of leaves from the fresh plant (or a heaped teaspoonful of the dried herb) in a cup, fill it with boiling water and infuse it, covered, for five to ten minutes. Lemon balm has a delicious lemony taste and it's not only good for your digestive system, it can also help calm the stress IBS sufferers so often feel.*

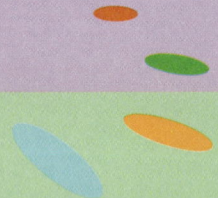

11

Dodge the Delhi belly

Everybody gets the runs sometimes, and over the centuries country folk have come up with a dozen different effective remedies.

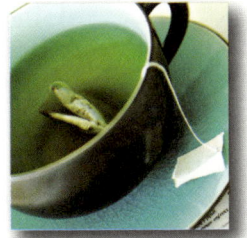

You may be surprised to learn that some of them can be found in your own kitchen, on the spice rack or in the fruit bowl.

There's diarrhoea and then there's diarrhoea. If the cramps are agonising, if there's blood in the watery stool you're passing, if you're nauseous or running a fever, seek medical help: you may be suffering an acute case of food-poisoning or worse.

Most cases of mild diarrhoea, though, don't need a doctor; it's your own body intelligently at work expelling wastes and impurities, such as that dodgy chemical-laden vino you keep pouring into it on holiday. And, for such cases, there are numbers of simple household remedies to turn to.

Who'd think of the prickly intrusive bramble as providing a cure? But when Elizabeth Janos travelled through New England and New York State questioning hundreds of older people about the country cures they remembered from their childhood, she found that dried blackberry roots were the number one remedy for diarrhoea. The roots were harvested in the autumn and dried. A handful of the

Here's an idea for you...

For fast first aid, try ordinary black or green tea. Make it nice and strong, let it cool a little, then drink three to four cups, without milk, over the day. Tea is rich in healing and soothing tannins.

dried roots was simmered in water until the liquid turned brownish black, and was then given by the cupful. In her book *Country Folk Medicine*, she quotes one woman who suffered from 'nervous bowels' as a child: 'My folks would boil blackberry roots and the tea would bind me right up.' Blackberry root was also the chief ingredient in one herbal remedy that my family relied on for years – the aptly named Spanish Tummy Mixture made up by the old-fashioned herbal firm Potters.

The root works well because it is full of nice astringent tannins to firm things up again, and soothe irritation and inflammation. Blackberry leaves have the same useful astringents, too. Both the powdered root and the dried leaves can be ordered from a herbal supplier to make a useful medicine-chest standby. To make a tea, take 2–3 teaspoons of the dried leaves or 1–2 teaspoons of the powdered root and add 250ml of boiling water. Steep for ten to fifteen minutes and drink up to three cups a day. Even the fruit itself can work a treat: try a cupful of the berries simmered till they just begin to yield their juice.

Dried bilberries or blueberries (they are close relatives, sharing the same properties) are another helpful fruit; an old European cure for diarrhoea was chewing dried bilberries. Since you can buy packets of dried blueberries in supermarkets these days, it might be a good idea to keep some in hand. They contain not only tannins but also pectin, a soluble fibre which will help bulk out the watery stools of diarrhoea and soothe the inflamed and irritated gut. Take 1–2 teaspoons at a time, chewing them very slowly and thoroughly up to three times a day. And, if you have nothing else in the house, a spoonful or so of blueberry or blackberry jelly, added to a small glass of hot water, might work a treat.

The root of the little yellow-flowered tormentil, *Potentilla tormentilla*, is especially high – up to 30% – in those wonder-working tannins. In the Swiss A. Vogel remedy for diarrhoea or irritable bowel syndrome, Tormentil Complex, the fresh root of tormentil is combined with oats, *Avena sativa*, which not only help calm irritated gut walls, but work to soothe the whole nervous system.

Another old European fruit cure is the common apple, grated raw and unpeeled (so use organically grown apples) or sliced and cooked into a light purée. Apples are rich in pectin, too. And, like blackberries and blueberries, they also supply plenty of the vital minerals, including potassium, which are lost in diarrhoea. And there's yet another item from the kitchen medicine chest: carrots grated and cooked to a very thin unsalted purée, a remedy you can even give to babies. Carrots are uniquely nourishing and soothing to the whole intestinal tract. But please, go for organically grown carrots – most supermarkets stock them these days.

'I look upon it that he who does not mind his belly will hardly mind anything else.'
JAMES BOSWELL, *The Life of Samuel Johnson*

Defining idea...

45

How did it go?

Q   **Someone told me that flax seeds are helpful in diarrhoea. How do they work?**

A   *Flax seeds, also known as linseeds, are loaded with mucilage, nice slippery stuff which relieves diarrhoea by soothing the gut lining, but also swelling in the digestive tract to help bulk out stools – an action as helpful in diarrhoea as it is in constipation. Linseeds are also a wonderful source of the famous omega-3 fatty acids currently hitting the health headlines. Look for an organic brand of ready-crushed seeds and take a tablespoonful, swallowing with at least 250ml of water – a good tumbler – to each tablespoonful. They need the water to swell inside you.*

Q   **My grandmother used to drink a lot of meadowsweet tea, and she told us it was good for anything wrong 'down there'. Is that a fact?**

A   *I don't know about 'anything', but this common wild flower is certainly great for diarrhoea. It reduces excess acidity, protects and heals the irritated gut, and soothes away pain. It's often combined with agrimony, another mild astringent. Put a dessertspoonful of the dried flowers and leaves (from a herbal supplier) in a cup, fill it with boiling water, cover and infuse for ten minutes, then strain and drink. Repeat two or three times a day.*

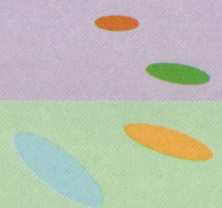

12

Bunged up

Huge numbers of people in Western-style societies suffer from chronic constipation.

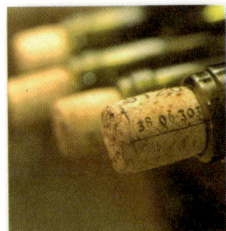

And for many of them, popping a laxative pill — 'helps keep you regular' — is as much part of their daily routine as brushing their teeth.

If you're eating a diet of highly refined and processed food – white flour, sugar, rice, pasta – and little or no fruit and veg, or nuts and seeds, it won't supply enough fibre to bulk out your stools for easy passage. And if you aren't drinking plenty of water, there won't be enough of it to add softness and bulk to your stools. Either way, they will be hard, dry and – quite literally – a pain in the ass. Making his TV series *Jamie's School Dinners*, celebrity chef Jamie Oliver was staggered to discover how many schoolkids were severely constipated on their diet of junk food.

If you're desk-bound and loathe exercise you'll have problems too: the muscles in your gut walls that keep things moving will have lost tone and elasticity. If you've been bombarding them with laxatives, which mostly work by irritating the gut wall into activity, then they may just forget how to work on their own. And finally, if you

Here's an idea for you...

Coffee can be very irritating to the whole digestive tract, and it's not a very good idea if you are constipated. Try dandelion coffee: it has a mildly laxative action, and it's a wonderful tonic for the whole digestive system.

don't go when you feel the urge – not just occasionally, but regularly – then the urge, too, may stop working. And then you're constipated, joining the sad millions who take the morning paper into the loo and sit grunting and straining for minutes on end.

If your case of constipation has come on out of the blue without any special changes in your diet, if it's painful or if it's been going on for more than a week, check it out with your doctor. But even 'normal' constipation should be a cause of concern. Bodily wastes are not meant to hang around in the colon for days at a time, stagnating, putrefying, and releasing toxins back into the body.

To get things moving again, there are two great herbal remedies: flax seeds (linseeds) or psyllium – the little dark seeds of plantain. Taken dry with plenty of water, both swell into a soft mass in your gut that not only helps produce bulky stools, but soothes and heals down under, and helps nudge lazy gut-wall muscles into action again. Look for a good brand and start with a teaspoon each morning, well-crushed and swallowed down with a full glass of water. After a week or so, add another teaspoon last thing at night. Finally, double the morning dose – and use even more water. The water is very important; without it the seeds could pile up to cause a bit of a blockage. You can buy flax seeds ready crushed.

Herbalist Dee Atkinson of Napier's makes up a mix of equal parts of psyllium seeds and the intriguingly-named slippery elm powder – the dried inner bark of an elm tree – and suggests to her patients that they sprinkle it onto their breakfast cereal.

Or take a couple of teaspoons three times a day, drinking plenty of water at the same time. Slippery elm is wonderfully soothing to an irritated gut, and has a useful antiseptic action too.

'Nearly the entire race is afflicted with constipation. Waste matter is left fermenting too long in the body.'
JETHRO KLOSS, *Back to Eden*

Defining idea...

There are a number of powerful herbal laxatives, such as cascara, aloes, rhubarb or buckthorn, or the senna which appears in dozens of different forms on any chemist's shelves. But most of them work by irritating the gut wall into action, and taking them is counterproductive in the long run, since your body will 'forget' how to operate properly without them. Keep them for the occasional emergency. For obstinate or chronic constipation, consult a herbalist, who will know how to blend these active agents with other herbs that can offset some of the damage they can cause unaided, and help tone and nourish the digestive system.

'The best herbal laxative is food,' remarks Herefordshire herbalist Christopher Robbins, in his book *The Household Herbal*. If you're a regular laxative-pill-popper, taper the dose off very slowly. At the same time start increasing your daily intake of fibre, but do it little by little. Think fibre-rich foods like dried fruit, nuts, seeds, fruit, vegetables. Eat wholemeal bread instead of white, jacket potatoes instead of mash, porridge instead of soggy cornflakes.

How did it go?

Q **I get constipated very easily, and I've noticed that it often coincides with really bad indigestion. Is there a connection, and what can I do about it?**

A *A sluggish digestive system can contribute to constipation and bitter herbs like dandelion can help. Herbalist Penelope Ody suggests this formula, in which the yellow dock has a gentle laxative action. You can order all the ingredients from a herbal supplier, mix it in the proportions given here, and make a day's supply at a time. You'll need 10g dried dandelion, 5g dried yellow dock root, 5g dried liquorice root and 5g dried anise seeds. Put them all in a pan, add 750ml of water, bring to the boil and simmer until the volume is reduced by a third. Pour into a jug, cool, and take a wineglass dose three times a day before meals.*

Q **I love coffee but I notice that when I drink a lot of it my constipation seems to get much worse. Are there any nice-tasting herbal teas I can have instead?**

A *Try fennel seed tea, which has a slightly sweet aniseed-like taste: it's an excellent after-meals tea as it helps settle the digestion. Elderflowers are mildly laxative, and make a delicious tea. Both are available in teabags. Lemon balm, which is very easy to grow, not only has a pleasant lemony taste but will also help sort out the nervous stomach that may be contributing to your constipation.*

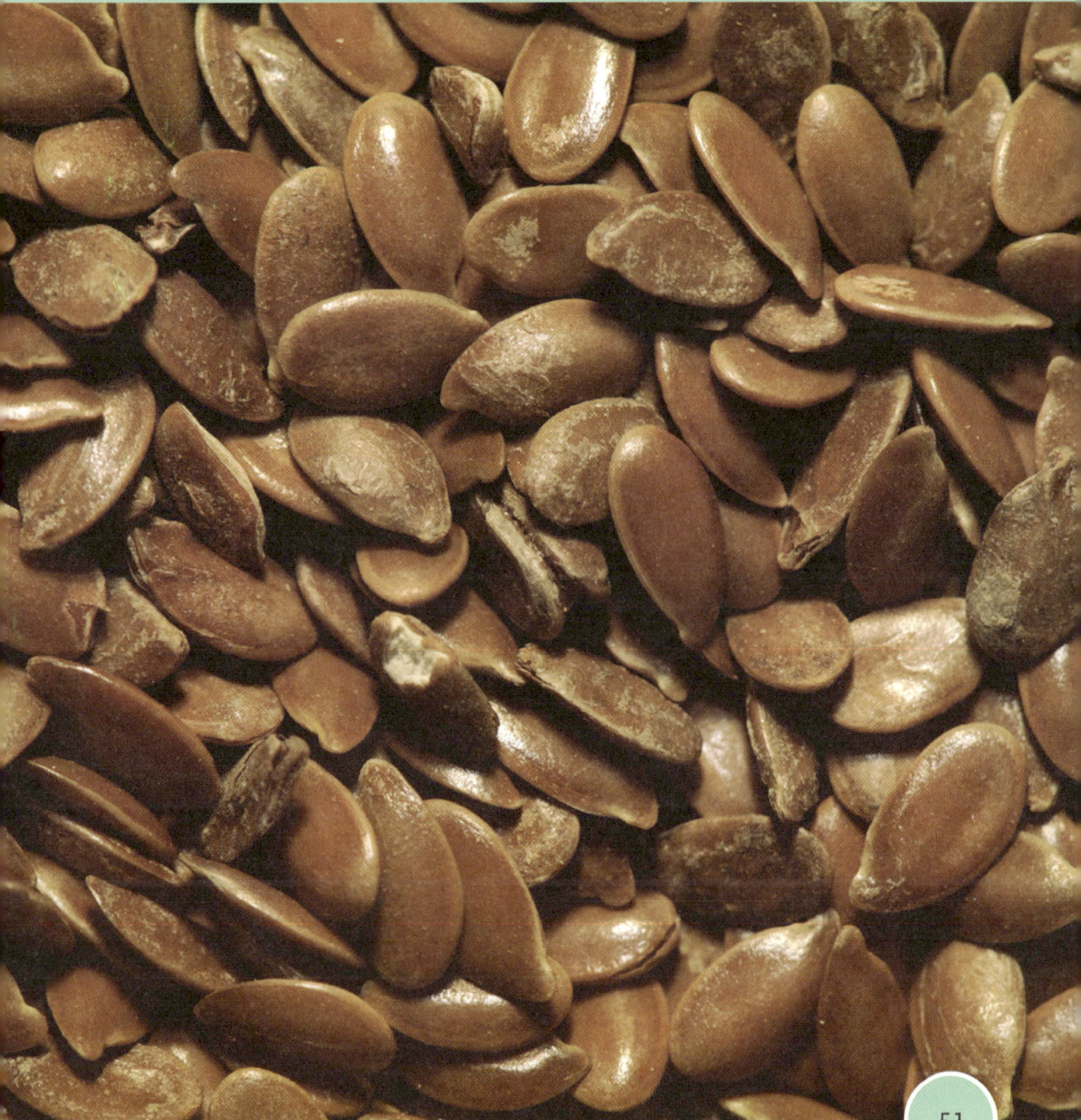

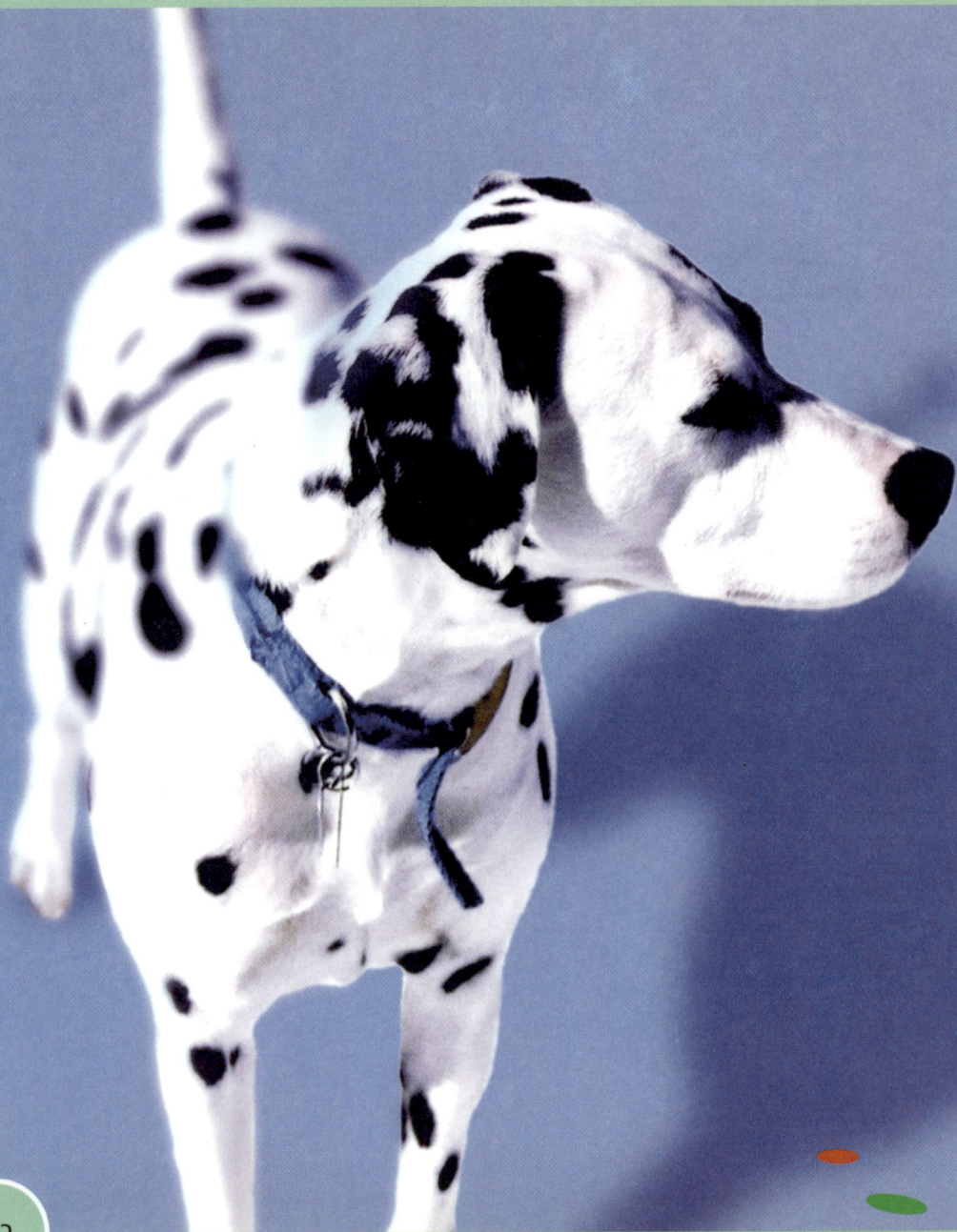

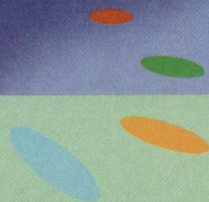

13

Damned spots

Cuts, scrapes, grazes, sores, burns and scalds are the commonest reason for raiding the first-aid kit.

But you can't beat herbal remedies for fast relief and healing.

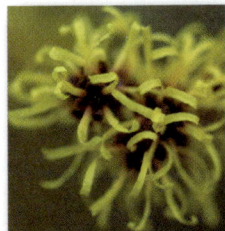

There are so many fantastic healing herbs that you could be stumped for choice. My own personal favourite is marigold, the hot-orange flower with the floppy pale green leaves, usually sold as calendula. I'm never without both the ointment and the tincture, and in my family we get through industrial quantities of both. Nothing seems to faze it.

When my daughters had their ears pierced, I didn't bother with surgical spirit when the new holes became infected, as they often did: I just applied a dot of pale yellow calendula ointment. Hey, presto! Instant pain relief and almost instant healing.

For the messy grazes, cuts, scrapes of daily childhood life, just clean carefully with warm water to which you add a dash of calendula tincture, then soothe calendula ointment over them and cover with a plaster. Calendula not only calms pain and inflammation and speeds healing, but it also counters infection – so you can also use it for minor cuts, or wounds that turn nasty.

Here's an idea for you...

Hard knocks can produce painful bruises, which show up as blood rushes to the site under the skin. To relieve the pain fast, apply ice-cold compresses of distilled witch hazel, renewing them until the pain has subsided. Witch hazel is a North American shrub, and the distilled preparation is on sale cheaply at any chemist. I find it an essential herb and keep a bottle cold in the fridge.

Comfrey is another amazing healing plant: it reduces pain and swelling rapidly. How does it work? Well, scientists finally figured out that a compound in comfrey called allantoin is the healer; it actually speeds healing by encouraging the production of new cells. Use comfrey ointment for nasty grazes but clean them thoroughly first, because the healing action of this wonder plant is so rapid that pus or dirt might become trapped inside. Comfrey can also be very effective for wounds that are slow to heal, such as bedsores. Not for nothing, incidentally, was comfrey once nicknamed 'bruise wort' by country people: it's a wonderful remedy for bruises. Apply the gel or ointment as soon as possible.

Another excellent remedy for bruises is the lovely Swiss mountain flower arnica. Apply the tincture – which should be diluted one part to five of water – or else use a ready-made ointment or gel from the health-food shop. (Caution: Arnica should never be applied where the skin is broken, and don't take it internally.)

Yet another great skin-healing agent is tea-tree oil, from Australia, one of the rare essential oils that can be applied direct to the skin. The common antiseptic Dettol was based on this oil, which is effective against viruses, bacteria and fungal infections alike. It doesn't sting, it eases pain and it boosts local circulation to speed healing. Wash cuts or sores then apply neat tea-tree oil. Very rarely, ultra-sensitive skin may become irritated by it, however.

A friend rang me to say that her mother was deeply depressed because the wounds left after a mastectomy operation were refusing to heal. The hospital had tried everything. I suggested she asked her nearest health-food store for a tube of ManukaCare 18 specially sterilised for hospital use. Manuka is a New Zealand plant and the bees feasting on its pollen produce a honey with extraordinary antibacterial powers. ManukaCare 18 – a specially sterilised form for medical purposes – certainly worked for my friend's mother. Manuka honey is increasingly being used in hospitals to treat badly infected ulcers, mastectomy wounds and bedsores resistant to antibiotics. It is even proving effective against the dreaded superbug...

'Nothing is really healed outside of us. The skin is only indicative of what is going on inside us.'
ROBYN KIRBY, Australian herbalist

Defining idea...

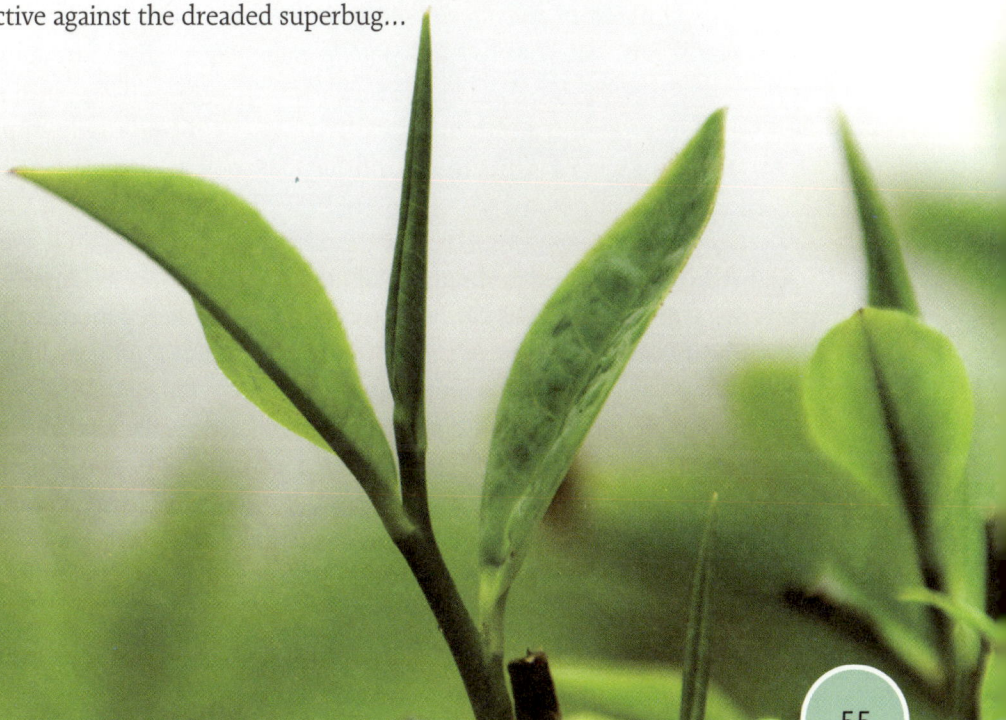

55

How did it go?

Q **Are there any good herbal remedies for burns?**

A *A really bad burn needs urgent medical attention, but minor burns, scalds or ordinary sunburn can be dealt with effectively by herbs. Don't forget that the first priority is to cool the area by spraying or soaking it with cold water. On holiday in Spain my son-in-law got painfully sunburnt on his shoulders: we found an aloe vera plant, hacked off a fat fleshy leaf, sliced it open, and applied the gooey, green, jelly-like inside directly to his reddened shoulders. The pain eased off and there were no blisters. In the US, the kitchen staff of many restaurants keep a big tube of aloe vera gel handy to deal with scalds, and one is an essential in my home first-aid kit. So is a bottle of lavender essential oil: it can be applied directly to burns and scalds, and it will soothe pain immediately.*

Q **My ten-year-old daughter is always chewing her nails, and often develops very painful pus-filled abscesses as a result. Can you suggest something to heal these quickly?**

A *It's calendula to the rescue. Fill an eggcup with plain water which is as hot as she can bear, and get her to soak her finger in it for ten to fifteen minutes; refresh the eggcup with more hot water during this time. Sometimes the pus can be pressed out after a few minutes; the hot water will make this easier. If it cannot, then put some calendula ointment on a plaster, wrap it firmly round her finger, and repeat next morning. Once the pus is all out, keep the finger clean and covered in a plaster with calendula ointment on it for a further day.*

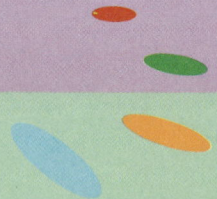

14

Scratching the itch

Eczema claims growing numbers of victims every year in the Western world.

You don't have to be one of them.

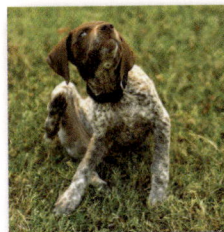

Let's get one thing straight, though: your cure is unlikely to come from conventional medicine. The steroid creams your doctor prescribes may ease the agony in the short term. Long term, they'll thin and damage the skin. Antihistamine pills may damp down the itching, but they often come with a price tag: side effects. Herbalists aim to get to the root of the problem, and then use herbs as effective treatment, both inside and skin-side. And, since sorting out and controlling eczema is a job for the long haul, it's encouraging to have a professional herbalist's advice and support along the way.

'When patients come in with really bad inflamed eczema,' says herbalist Dee Atkinson, 'the first thing to do is to calm it down, so I prescribe calming herbs such as chamomile, oats or nettle, either in tea or tincture form. You can buy some herbs in juiced form, which is yet another way to take them. Most of my patients are on steroid creams when they first come to see me. I give them some starflower cream, and encourage them to mix it with their steroid cream: put a blob of each in the palm of their hand, and blend them before applying. Then gradually reduce the amount of steroid cream they are using. Starflower cream – alternatively called borage cream – really takes the itch out of eczema.'

Here's an idea for you...

A cream made from marigold flowers, also known as calendula cream, can be a wonderful ally. Apply it freely to all the reddened, itchy bits, and soothe it well in; it helps pain and calms inflammation. Since it's also antifungal and antibacterial, it can also protect your skin against the secondary infections so easily set up in scratched or weepy skin. Herbalist Sue Eldin finds it a highly successful treatment. 'The more frequently it is applied and the better it is rubbed into the skin, the greater the improvement,' she says.

Stress is a huge factor in eczema: a friend's face once broke out literally as she was given news of her daughter's serious illness, she told me later. There are numbers of herbs that can help calm down and deal with whatever is stressing you – skullcap, chamomile, passionflower, lemon balm, limeflower and lavender among them. You'll find most of these used in ready-blended herbal teas aimed at particular ailments, such as stress or anxiety. One immediate practical step you can take is to cut down on caffeine and alcohol, and drink plenty of these natural calmers.

Many cases of eczema come from inside. Your body could be reacting to chemicals in your environment and taking it out – literally – on your skin. Small babies often develop eczema because they're reacting to the cows' milk in their formula.

Sue Eldin, a medical herbalist working within a conventional medical practice in London, fingers another suspect: chemical additives. With four to ten year olds, she notes, a lot of the foods, drinks and snacks aimed at this young market are highly coloured and highly flavoured. 'In all cases, when these foods are replaced with realistic alternatives, the severity of the eczema decreases.' To identify other triggers, Sue gets her patients to turn detective. For a week, they keep a double-entry food diary.

On one side they note each day's intake of any food, drink or drug, and the time it was consumed; on the opposite page, they record flare-ups or aggravations, with a note of the time. Matching flare-ups to a specific food or drink is often straightforward, and patients avoid it thereafter.

'Happiness is having a scratch for every itch.'
OGDEN NASH

Defining idea...

Baby – and adult – skin can also be acutely sensitive to the dozens of dodgy chemicals in laundry products, bathroom and skin care toiletries. Replace them with the 'green' products now available, based on plants and natural oils, and you may find your skin responds with a delightful improvement.

Four common weeds crop up all the time in herbal prescriptions for eczema: dandelion, burdock, nettle and red clover. Dandelion nourishes the liver to help boost excretion of wastes: eat the peppery young leaves in salads or stews. Burdock, a great blood-cleanser, is a traditional remedy for a whole slew of skin problems, calming inflammation and protecting the skin from bacterial infection. Mineral-rich nettles and red clover are reliable blood cleansers too, and nettles also supply natural antihistamines, to help quell the allergic reactions which may be triggering your eczema.

Why all this fuss about cleansing? Because it's reckoned that as much as a quarter of the body's wastes are excreted through the skin. So herbalists will prescribe herbs that help along the whole cleansing process to give your skin a break. You can take regular doses of any of these four herbs in the form of a tincture. Follow the manufacturer's directions for dosage, and persevere for at least a month.

How did it go?

Q   **Is there something really soothing I can put in my bath to calm that awful hot, itchy feeling?**

A   *Try oatmeal. Stuff the toe of a nylon stocking – or one half of a pair of tights – with ordinary oatmeal, then tie the stocking round the bath tap so that your bath water flows through it. The oatmeal will turn the water milky, and it's very soothing. Keep the bath temperature warm, rather than hot.*

Q   **My poor skin is so horribly dry. Is there a good herbal moisturiser I can use?**

A   *Eczema-afflicted skin is dry skin, and in some cases it can be caused by a lack of nourishing fatty acids. The seeds of the striking yellow evening primrose and the furry blue borage that looks so pretty in your Pimms both supply one of these. They can be taken in capsule form. You need the omega-3 essential fatty acids too, and freshly ground linseeds (also called flax seeds) are another great source: grind them and eat them on cereal, or sprinkled on salads or by the spoonful, washed down with plenty of water, to keep your skin well-nourished from within.*

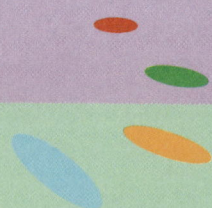

15

Pimpled youth

Tried everything for that face full of zits? The antibiotics, the dodgy vitamin-A derivatives, the contraceptive pill, the chemical peels? And nothing worked long term?

Don't despair: herbal medicine is full of great options for an acne cure.

Hormonal mayhem can be a big acne trigger, with the male hormone testosterone fingered as the chief suspect. This is likely to be especially true for stressed teenagers, or for women suffering PMS (a lot of women see it vanish for ever with the birth of their first baby – as in my case). The herb chastetree – *Vitex agnus castus* – can help women rebalance those troublesome hormones, often sorting out PMS problems as a nice side effect. A herbalist can fine-tune a personal prescription for you, giving you good advice about diet and lifestyle at the same time.

Professional herbalists like to work at skin problems from the inside out. They point out that your body offloads its rubbish through the skin as well as through the bladder, rectum and lungs. So they swear by a handful of herbs to carry out some internal cleansing.

Two of the most important are common countryside weeds – dandelion and burdock. You can take them in the form of a tea, or as an easy-to-take tincture, made from the roots of either – or, better still, both. As with all herbal acne treatments, you'll need to persevere; in this case for at least a month.

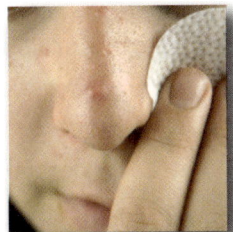

Here's an idea for you...

Can't stop picking at those horrid pimples? Keep handy a bottle of calendula tincture, made from gorgeous marigolds. If you've scratched your pimples into open weeping sores, clean them up with a damp cotton wool ball onto which you sprinkle a few drops of calendula. It's fabulous stuff – antiseptic, soothing, healing. Alternatively, try tea-tree oil, and apply it neat to spots with a cotton wool bud. Patch-test first, though. In a clinical trial carried out in Australia, sufferers found it worked just as well as benzoyl peroxide but without the stinging, burning and redness.

Another herb, wild pansy (*Viola tricolor*), is considered by herbalists as practically specific for acne. You can buy it in tincture form, often combined with other cleansing and helpful herbs such as nettle, cleavers, dandelion and red clover.

Tinctures, alcoholic extracts of herbs, are a great way to make the herbal medicine go down, incidentally. Order from a reliable herbal supplier, and follow the dosage directions: you simply dropper the right amount into a glass of water. But no one suffering the shame and embarrassment of acne will be content just to swallow stuff. You'll want to be actively targeting those pits and pustules. Here are some suggestions.

Ordinary face-masks can be pretty rough on the skin. Try one made from green clay powder, sold at health-food stores. You'll need 2 tablespoons of the powder. Add the juice of half a lemon, 3–5 drops of tea-tree oil, 3–5 drops of lemon essential oil and enough water to make a paste. Spread it on the affected bits, leave for fifteen minutes, wash off with tepid water and then spray your face with healing, calming lavender water.

Lemon juice on its own can help dry out and heal the pimples: paint them with freshly squeezed juice at bedtime, leave on overnight, then rinse off in the morning. Herbal tea bags can also be easy first aid. Make up a cuppa of chamomile or yarrow tea, let it cool, then keep it in the fridge and use it as a cleansing face tonic. Herbal infusions should be used within a day; to save a lot of brewing, freeze a two-tea-bag dose in an ice-cube tray, then defrost a couple of cubes as and when you need them.

'Adolescence is just one big walking pimple.'
CAROL BURNETT, American actor and comedian

Defining idea...

Don't wash your face! No amount of scrubbing with soap and water is going to remove those wretched zits; you'll just end up with bone-dry skin. Why? Because your skin has its own protective coating, a sheen of fine oil secreted non-stop by millions of tiny glands. This coating doesn't just keep your skin moist. It also fights off harmful bugs. Washing swipes it off, as do harsh cleansers and alcohol-based toning lotions. The best alternative may surprise you: it's an oil. Virgin coconut oil, to be precise: a white wax that liquefies as it warms. Use it as a cleanser and make-up remover at night; apply it all over your face, then gently tissue off to leave your skin smooth and soft. In the morning, give your face a cold splash, then re-apply just a touch of coconut oil. There are anecdotal accounts of acne yielding to just weeks of the coconut treatment.

How did it go?

Q I'm in my early thirties, my acne is finally gone, but my face is still covered with scars. I use concealer all the time, but they don't seem to be fading at all. Can you help?

A *Relax – at your age my skin was just as scarred from years of acne. But five to ten years after the last zit vanished, the scars had all faded. And I didn't even know about amazing Rosa mosqueta oil. This pale yellow miracle comes from the seeds of a wild rose growing high in the Chilean Andes. Applied regularly, the oil has an extraordinary ability to rehabilitate damaged skin, smoothing away even stretch marks and surgical scarring. Incidentally, save that concealer stick for special occasions – and leave your skin free to get on with healing itself the rest of the time. Use Rosa mosqueta cream as a daily moisturiser, too.*

Q My dermatologist says diet has nothing to do with acne. Is this right?

A *Not necessarily. You may be sensitive to certain foods, and the reaction shows up in your skin. I once had a Dutch au pair who had frightful acne. She also drank about a gallon of coffee a day, and got through startling amounts of her favourite Gouda cheese. When she was finally persuaded to cut right back on both, her acne cleared slowly but surely, and was gone for good within six months.*

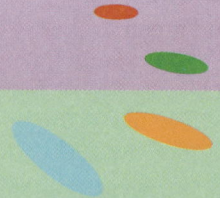

16

Detox and thrive

Detoxing: who needs it?

Answer: every single one of us. We need detoxing so badly that our bodies are actually hard at it 24/7, 365 days a year, without a break.

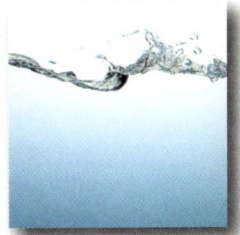

You know you need a spot of extra detoxing if you're tired, if you have big bags under your eyes, if you feel headachey, if you're constipated, if your periods are a real pain, if your stools are smelly and your breath not-so-fresh, if your eye-whites aren't white and your tongue is heavily coated.

Just what does all this detoxing remove? It's the normal wastes created in-house by day-to-day living, plus the toxic polluting chemicals we take in with our food, our drink and even the air we breathe or fill our homes with in cleaning, cosmetic and toiletry products.

Start by cutting down on the toxic load: alcohol, nicotine, coffee, fizzy drinks, too much sweet, fatty, additive-loaded food and household or cosmetic chemicals. Drink six to eight glasses of water – preferably filtered – every day. And discover a team of herbs that have been used for centuries for cleansing and detox. In medieval times, country people would make up 'spring drinks' from herbs sprouting young, fresh and green in the hedgerows – dandelion, nettles and that sticky, clinging stuff

Here's an idea for you...

The French obsess about the health of their livers, and if you eat in any French bistro in the springtime, you will find their favourite dandelion salad on the menu: salade de pissenlit. Snippets of bacon are fried until crisp, a little vinegar is swished around the pan, and then its contents are poured over a dish of the sharp-tasting fresh young leaves. A very enjoyable way to do your liver a bit of good.

cleavers. After a winter diet of stodge and salted or dried foods, these spring drinks supplied a badly needed boost of tonic and cleansing phytochemicals. 'A course of dandelion treatment in the spring,' wrote the modern French herb enthusiast Jean Palaiseul, 'will tone up your whole body, cleansing it of the waste matter deposited by the heavy clogging food of winter.'

Much of your body's garbage ends up in your urine, filtered by your kidneys. Nettles stimulate both kidney and bladder function, and they're rich in cleansing, nourishing minerals too. Both dandelion and nettle come high on any herbalist's list of cleansing, detoxing herbs today.

Cleavers boosts the efficiency of your lymphatic system, that efficient drainage network that helps remove toxins from the body, and it's good news for the skin too. Herbalists include it in prescriptions for acne, eczema and psoriasis, as well as arthritis and gout.

Croatian herbalist Dragana Vilinac formulates herbal blends and tinctures for one of the UK's most popular herbal suppliers. And when I asked her to suggest an effective mix of detox herbs, I was not surprised to find both dandelion and nettle in it, as well as burdock – 'an esteemed blood cleanser and digestive stimulant,' she explains. Here's her formula: burdock root, 5g; dandelion root, 5g; nettle root, 5g.

Put them in a pan with 600ml of water, bring to the boil, cover the pan and simmer very gently for fifteen to twenty minutes. Take it off the heat, leave to steep for another fifteen minutes, then strain and drink a small mugful three times daily. This trio of roots, she explains, will enhance the elimination of wastes, help offload toxic wastes and calm any inflammation. Stock up with the ingredients from a herbal supplier, and give yourself a two-week course, cutting down on caffeine, alcohol and junk food at the same time, and drinking plenty of water.

'Health is not a "gift" but something each person is responsible for through his or her own daily effort.'
HIDEO NAKAYAMA, Japanese dermatologist

Defining idea...

Dragana also suggests another version, for occasional use, which is quicker and easier to prepare. Leaves are milder medicine than roots, so: dandelion leaf, 5g; nettle leaf, 5g; cleavers, 5g. 'This will help protect the body from the accumulation of excess fluid around the waist, under the skin, in the lungs in the form of phlegm, in the bladder,' she says. To brew it, mix the herbs, put 2 teaspoons in a mug of boiling water, steep for ten minutes, strain and drink.

Nettles, cleavers and dandelion can all be gathered wild in the spring but make sure they haven't been sprayed, either with pesticides or by a passing dog. Pick only the youngest and freshest ones, and eat them lightly steamed.

In German folk medicine, the seeds of the impressive milk thistle were used for jaundice and other liver complaints. Modern researchers have found that it can actually protect and regenerate liver cells, good news for overworked, hungover livers. Take a ten-day course of it. Women on the contraceptive pill, or those who are pregnant or breastfeeding, should avoid it, though.

67

How did it go?

Q I always mean to start one of those post-Christmas detoxes when I'm feeling bunged up with too much food and drink. But I just don't feel like it when the weather is still all dark and miserable. Should I have a bit more willpower?

A *Definitely not. Newspapers and women's magazines all combine to plug the post-festive detox, but the coldest time of year is no time for this. Save it for the longer, lighter, more energetic days of spring. And drastic detoxing, by the way, is not for you if you have a serious medical condition, if you're taking prescribed medication, if you have liver or gallbladder problems – or if you're unwell, getting over the flu, pregnant, breastfeeding or over sixty.*

Q I feel a real mess, with a spotty skin, lank hair, and quite a few excess pounds. Can you suggest a great pick-me-up?

A *The leaves of the beautiful silver birch have always been a popular cleansing spring tonic in northern Europe. They're specially good at dealing with that heavy, bloated, lethargic sensation that winter often leaves behind. The young leaves are harvested fresh in the spring, and made into a juice or elixir that will really help shift that winter rubbish, and leave you feeling clearer and brighter.*

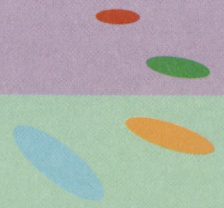

17

Mad dogs and Englishmen

Sunburn is the most easily avoided of all human woes.

But we still lie sprawled on tropical beaches in our millions, soaking up the lovely, deadly midday sun...

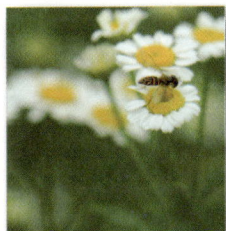

And by nightfall we suddenly realise that our bright pink skin is not just pre-tan: it's a nasty burn. Luckily, there are half a dozen herbal remedies which can bring near-instant relief; just don't go travelling to that sundrenched resort without at least one of them.

Top of the list is aloe vera, that fleshy-leaved cactus grown all over the Mediterranean as an ornamental plant. Slice through one of those fat leaves and you'll find a thick gel inside: apply it to a burn, and the relief is almost magical. Aloe vera soothes pain, calms inflammation, and speeds the healing process by stimulating the growth of new tissue. You can buy this wonder-working gel in tubes; no first-aid kit or kitchen cupboard should be without it.

In the case of severe burns – sunburn or any other kind – get professional help urgently to deal with the shock, dehydration and systemic infection that can result. But since it's the heat that's doing the damage, a first priority is to cool the burned area, if possible by immersing it in cold water or by keeping a stream of cool water running over it.

Here's an idea for you...

Chamomile is a great healer for sunburn. If there's nothing else handy on that beach, order plenty of chamomile tea from the beach bar, add ice cubes to cool it and apply it to the deep pink bits after you've showered.

Another great burns remedy is tincture of marigold. If most of you is sunburnt, soak in a cool bath to which you've added plenty of this – a good splash of it. When you emerge, apply compresses of cold water, to which you've added more marigold, to the worst bits and rest, lying down to keep the compresses in place.

Throughout history, honey has been revered as a healing remedy for wounds and injuries of every kind. And that includes burns. In a study reported in the *British Journal of Surgery* in 1991, the efficacy of honey as a treatment was compared with one of the standard medical treatments for minor burns, silver sulphadiazine cream. Most – 87% – of the patients treated with honey were healed within fifteen days, compared to only 10% in the silver sulphadiazine group.

The last thing you'd want to apply to a stinging burn, you might think, is anything like a stinging nettle. Not so, according to a British herbalist, the late John Evans, who in a herbal magazine told the story of how he treated his badly sunburnt daughter on holiday, when he had none of his usual tinctures and ointments to hand. By night-time her pain was so severe that she could not bear even a sheet over her. After searching the nearby lane by torchlight, he harvested an armful of nettles and dumped them in a panful of boiling water to make a pale green infusion. As soon as it had cooled, he laid pieces of linen soaked in the infusion on the sensitive sunburnt skin and within a few minutes the pain was subsiding. By the morning his daughter was perfectly comfortable and the angry red inflammation had completely disappeared. You can use a diluted tincture of nettle in the same way and you can buy a lotion that combines nettles with arnica flowers from a homeopathic range.

'I never expected to see the day when girls would get sunburned in places they now do.'
WILL ROGERS

Defining idea...

Don't forget, by the way, that any burn, other than the most minor, can be a severe shock to its victim. Treat that shock with a wonderful combination of flower essences, Dr Bach's Rescue Remedy.

The French chemist Robert Gattefosse was one of the founding fathers of aromatherapy – the healing power of essential oils. In the 1920s he burned his hand badly in a laboratory experiment, looked round for treatment and plunged the hand into a jar of pure lavender oil. The pain was gone in minutes, there were no blisters and no scarring, either. I tried the lavender oil treatment on a neighbour of mine when she picked up a frying-pan by a handle she hadn't realised was red hot. After holding her red and throbbing hand under a running cold tap till it cooled, I gently dried it with sterile lint, then poured a teaspoon of neat lavender oil onto the burned area. The relief astonished us both: a day later there was little sign of the nasty burn.

How did it go?

Q I've read research suggesting that standard suntan products may themselves be carcinogenic once the sun gets to them, and I don't like putting all those chemicals on my skin. Is there a good natural sunscreen?

A *Yes, says herbalist Peter Jackson-Main, jojoba oil: 'It has a natural SPF of around sixteen, and I have used nothing else for many years. Sunburn used to be routine for me with my fair northern skin: not any more. Add lavender oil for pleasant aroma and extra anti-burning action.' Jojoba oil is also rich in antioxidant vitamins, and a wonderful moisturiser for any skin type; it's not an essential oil, so you don't have to worry about applying it directly to your skin. Price-wise, even the best pure organic jojoba oil compares favourably with some of the pricier sunscreens.*

Q A bad scald recently left me with a nasty scar on my forearm. Any ideas for getting rid of it?

A *Soothe a little* Rosa mosqueta *oil into the scarred area every night. You should see a definite improvement quite soon. This oil, made from roses growing wild in the Andes, originally became known as an anti-wrinkle treatment, but Chilean researchers tested it on 180 patients with scars from injuries, burns or surgery, and discovered that it has unbelievable regenerative powers, restoring much of the skin's natural softness and texture. In another study, it reversed much of the damage done to complexions by long months spent at the beach. So give it a try.*

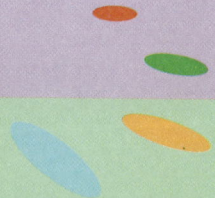

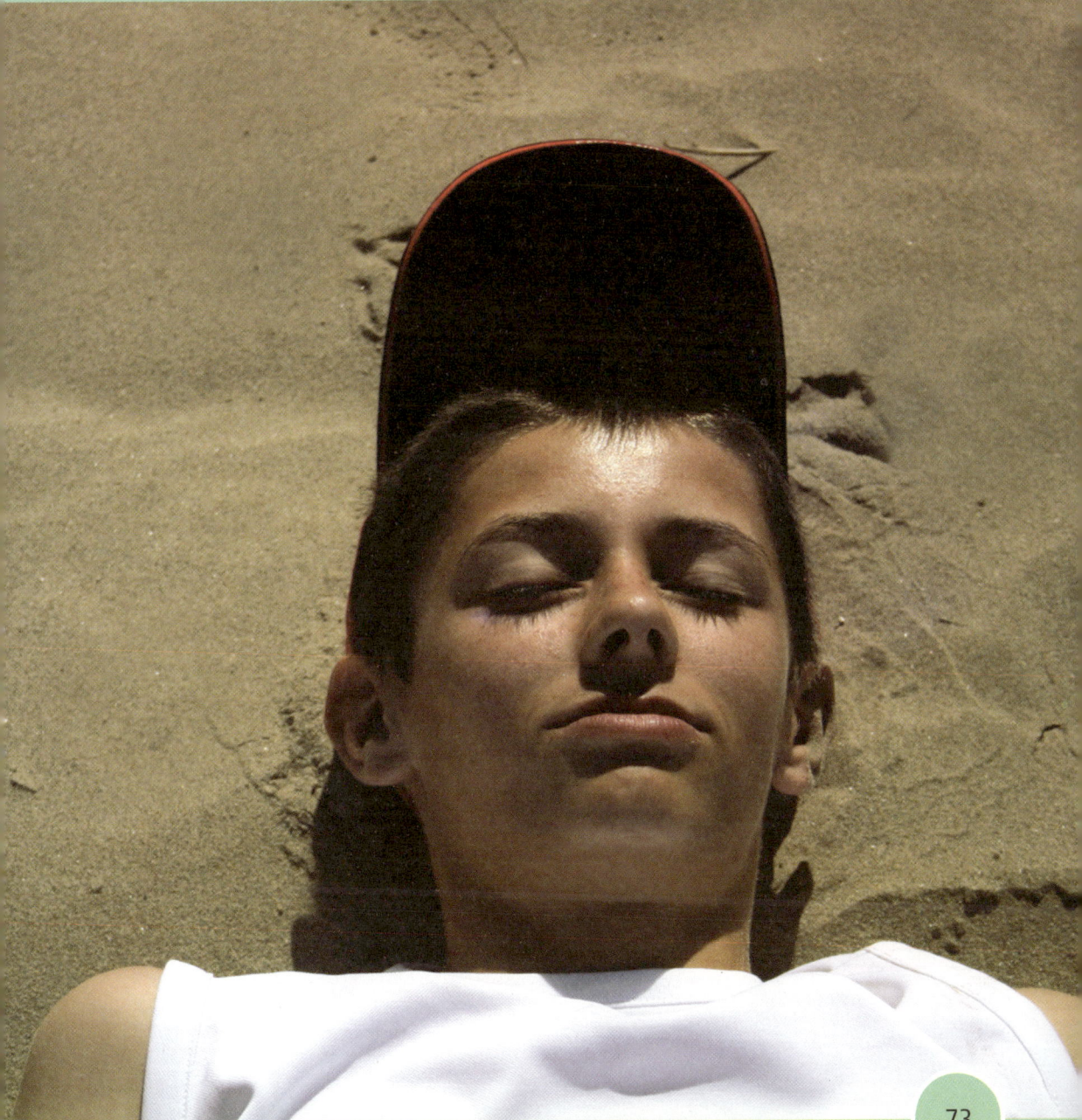

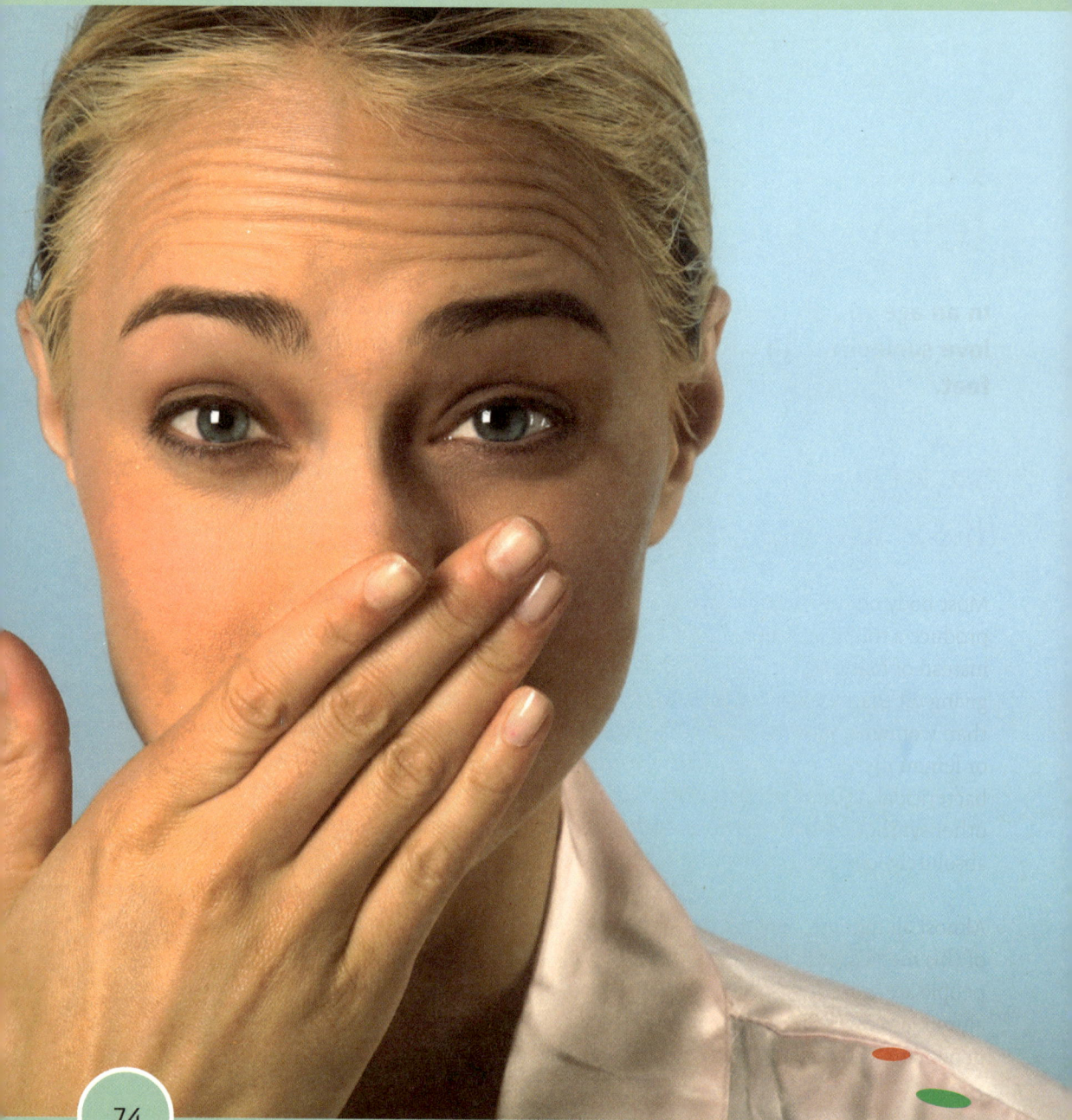

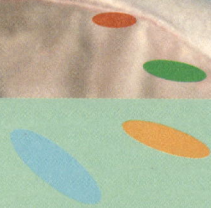

18

What your best friend won't tell you

In an age so painfully aware of body odours, it's hard to love someone with bad breath, rank underarms or smelly feet.

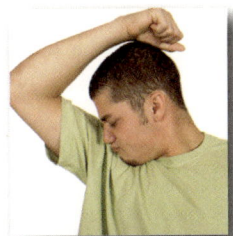

So let's take a look at some natural answers to these age-old problems.

Most body odour comes from under the arms, where the tiny apocrine glands produce a milky secretion. It doesn't smell bad to start with but if it hangs around, instead of being washed off regularly, bacteria will colonise it, multiply and start giving off that familiar old reek. Men have bigger and more active apocrine glands than women, and some people have overactive ones, too. Soaps with added tea tree or lemon myrtle, both from Australia, are fresh and pleasant-smelling as well as bactericidal. Wear clothes that let your skin breathe; nylon, acrylic, polyester and other synthetic fabrics create a close, warm, airless atmosphere that bacteria absolutely love and thrive in.

Almost all modern deodorants and antiperspirants are based on aluminium, because of this metal's drying qualities. But underarm skin is highly absorbent, and some people are worried about the build-up in our bodies of a foreign metal (excess aluminium has been linked with Alzheimer's). Instead, choose a plant-based deodorant. Sage is an obvious choice here: this great flavouring herb is not only an

Here's an idea for you...

In a study conducted by a French naturopath, Eric Nigelle, twenty-seven people afflicted by body odour – five of them severely so – tried out this lemon juice treatment over twelve months. Every morning, they applied 10 drops of freshly squeezed lemon juice to each armpit. Afterwards, twenty-five of them had no further problems, and the remaining two were much improved. Definitely worth a try.

efficient antiseptic, but it also has drying powers which make it useful in the treatment of night sweats and hot flushes, as well as common or garden perspiration. James Duke, a leading US authority on healing herbs, suggests using cider vinegar to swab underarms as an alternative, and suggests steeping several leaves of sage in it for a couple of weeks, to make it even more effective.

Sage is one of the chosen smells in a trio of brilliant deodorants from a great European range of bodycare products. They're made using only natural ingredients including herbal extracts to neutralise bacteria and a range of essential oils. The other two smells are citrus, and my favourite, wild rose, which contains essential oils known for their deodorising action – rose, ylang-ylang, geranium and neroli among them. It smells much too nice to be an effective deodorant, but in consumer trials its effect was found to last from five to nine hours. If your body odour persists despite all your efforts, see your doctor.

Bad breath is even less acceptable in our modern society than body odour and chewing pastilles or spraying oral deodorants into the problem mouth are short-term answers. You need to work out just why your breath is offensive and deal with that.

There are two possibilities. Firstly, trouble down in the gut, where the wastes of your last meal may be hanging around too long because of constipation. Digestive upsets or malfunction are a common cause of bad breath, and need to be sorted out. Another obvious cause is tooth problems: decaying teeth and gum pockets filled with busy bacteria producing malodorous gases. Take yourself off to your dentist, and steel yourself to learning good oral hygiene, then doing it regularly. Use a plant-based toothpaste featuring one of a trio of herbs with outstanding antiseptic qualities: tea tree, neem from India and propolis.

The mouthwashes available at most chemists are usually alcohol-based – very drying for the mouth – and packed with dodgy colouring and flavouring additives. Instead, go for a mouthwash based on natural antiseptics – neem, tea tree or propolis again. Tincture of propolis makes an excellent mouthwash too: add 10 drops to a couple of tablespoons of water, and swish it all around your mouth and teeth for a couple of minutes. A tea of sage, thyme or rosemary – use a teaspoon of the dried herb, a sprig or two of the fresh, infused for ten minutes, covered, in a cupful of boiling water – will be just as effective an antiseptic to excess micro-organisms. It will help tone and strengthen your gums into the bargain.

'Let your armpits be charm-pits...'
Well-known advertising slogan

Defining idea...

How did it go?

Q **My teenage son has startlingly smelly feet. He's quite self-conscious about them. Is there anything I can do to help?**

A *Reluctance to wash, ripe old socks being worn for days on end and cheap, airless trainers only cast off at bedtime are common causes of this problem. But in some cases even basic hygiene doesn't solve it, so here are some suggestions. Persuade your son to soak his feet at bedtime in a bowl of warm water to which you add a couple of spoonfuls of bicarbonate of soda plus a good splash of cider vinegar, or a few drops of tea-tree oil. Give him sage, rosemary or thyme tea, made as above, to swab his feet daily. And supply him with an antiseptic soap containing neem, tea tree or lemon myrtle.*

Q **I hate all those minty breath-fresheners – they just advertise the fact that you're insecure about your breath. Are there any great alternatives?**

A *At the end of a meal, Indians often chew on aromatic spices to help banish that waft of curry: cumin, fennel and cardamom seeds are favourites. Western alternatives feature the antiseptic and deodorant qualities of bright green chlorophyll in plants: chew parsley or fresh mint, a much nicer smell than those pastilles. All of these natural breath-fresheners, incidentally, are also excellent aids to digestion.*

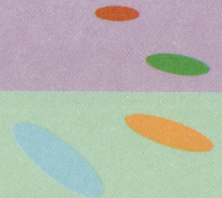

19

Ugh – unwelcome guests

From time to time low-life creatures such as head lice, amoebas, mites and intestinal worms opt for an easy life in our hair, in our guts or just under our skin.

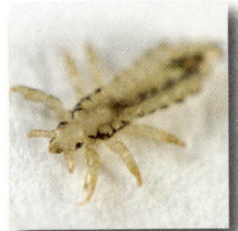

And they're trouble.

But you don't always need powerful chemicals to get rid of them: some natural and herbal alternatives can be just as effective.

One of the worst horrors is the scabies mite which (once having reached you through close physical contact with another victim) burrows happily into your skin, causing a maddening itchy red rash. Favoured spots are between fingers and toes, armpits, the genital area and the wrists. The orthodox treatment is by the application of powerful insecticides, including organophosphates which have largely been banned from agricultural use because of possible nervous-system damage. I, personally, would be unhappy about leaving myself coated overnight in such a toxic substance. Fortunately, there are excellent alternatives.

The leaves, seed and oil of the Indian neem tree have been used as safe natural insecticides for thousands of years. To treat infestations, apply neem oil, or a neem leaf and oil cream, to your whole body – especially bits where a red rash is already showing – and leave it on overnight. (Patch-test it on the skin first, though, in case

Here's an idea for you...

Dr Valnet, the Frenchman who virtually invented medical aromatherapy last century, suggests this cure for a parasitic infestation. Grate or crush 3–4 cloves of fresh garlic into a cupful of boiling water or milk. Let it steep all night. Strain it and drink it – fasting – the next morning, and repeat daily during the following three weeks.

of a reaction, and only use it externally.) The essential oil of lavender works extremely well against scabies, too, and smells more attractive. Patch-test first, as with neem, then stroke it in all over your body. You can add a few drops to a shampoo and wash your hair, as well.

You'll need to disinfect everything that has possibly been in contact with scabies. To do this, make up a pleasant-smelling disinfectant from 100ml of neat vodka, to which you add the following essential oils: 1 teaspoon of lavender oil, 25 drops of geranium and 20 of camphor. Use it to sponge bedding, upholstery, coat collars, etc.

A wide range of parasites can home in to take up residence inside you. These include tapeworms and nasties picked up in exotic holiday spots, and less alarming species such as the thread worm rampant among schoolchildren these days. Parasitic infections are becoming extremely common in this age of global travel, though many of them are home-grown too.

Prevention is much better than cure. Dr Alfred Vogel, the great Swiss naturopath and herbalist, travelled extensively in the tropics in search of new remedies for his patients. Some Amazonian Indians suggested he chew a leaf of the papaya plant to protect himself from the dangerous parasites – hookworms, amoebas and whip worms among them – that were rampant in the region. He followed their advice and was never troubled by parasitic infestation in all his travels. The leaves and unripe fruit of the papaya contain an enzyme, papain, which actually digests intestinal parasites in your gut. Cut down on meat, eggs and fish and take a bottle of papaya pills with you when you're travelling in exotic countries.

A number of common plants will make you a lot less attractive to parasites if you eat them regularly, such as garlic, carrots, lemons, fennel, parsley, leek, fresh pineapple and onions. Sugar, refined foods and alcohol, on the other hand, will greatly enhance your appeal to parasites.

Shelled pumpkin seeds have a long history of folk use for expelling worms. As occasional protection, grind a tablespoonful of them, add to a glass of carrot juice and take before breakfast, repeating the dose twice during the day. Or you can add them to your muesli. Mix with a cupful of water and soak overnight; by breakfast time they will be nice and chewy.

'Parasitism is the most popular animal lifestyle on the planet.'
KEVIN LAFFERTY, US research ecologist

Defining idea...

How did it go?

Q **My six-year-old son is very restless at night and scratches his bottom a lot. I suspect thread worms – is there a herbal cure?**

A *Try vampire medicine! Crush a little fresh garlic into a teaspoon of vaseline ointment and smear it around his anus last thing at night. Then wash his bottom first thing in the morning. Do this for a fortnight and you'll break the cycle of infestation and kill off the little beasts. If you – or he – hates the smell, use a couple of drops of tea-tree or eucalyptus oil in the ointment instead.*

Q **I'm tired of combing through my eleven-year-old daughter's hair for head lice, and the delousing shampoos smell really horrid. Any herbal answers?**

A *Those delousing lotions are made from highly toxic organophosphate pesticides, so you're right to be unenthusiastic about applying them to a child's head. Instead, you could try neem oil, though you may not like the smell of that much, either, and tea-tree oil is also death to lice, so give that a go. Add a teaspoonful of neem or tea-tree oil to a tablespoonful of olive oil and comb it through the hair as before. Leave it for ten minutes and then shampoo with a tea-tree shampoo before nit-combing. The treatment can be repeated as often as necessary – but patch-test the oil on the skin before applying them to the scalp. There are specially formulated neem or tea-tree delousing shampoos too.*

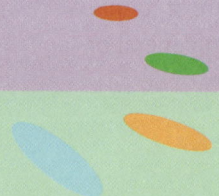

20

Not tonight, Josephine...

Impotence is most men's worst nightmare: the problem they hate to talk about, even to their doctors.

The more they obsess about it, too, the worse it gets.

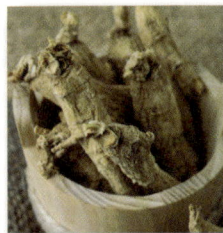

However, the massive research prompted by the runaway success of Viagra has made one thing clear: impotence – or erectile dysfunction, ED for short, as it is now known – is certainly not all in the mind. ED can result from one of a number of glitches in the reproductive system, as well as problems such as diabetes or kidney disease. So you should discuss libido or erectile problems with your doctor in order to rule out a physiological cause.

'There's a general belief,' says UK herbalist Peter Conway, 'that herbs may have something to offer men with potency problems' – and he sees quite a lot of them. 'Impotence has many factors,' he points out, 'and in my experience the commonest ones are stress and fatigue. Most of the guys I've seen are tired. They're working very hard, not eating very well, probably skipping breakfast, and anxious about their sexual performance – anxious generally. Most of them aren't getting enough sleep. Sleep and diet are key factors. I get them to eat a decent wholefood diet, ask them about exercise, how they relax.'

'Depression can really affect performance: three herbs I use most often in such cases are St John's wort, borage and skullcap. And if anxiety is the problem – about stuff in general or sexual performance in particular – valerian is usually reliable.

The well-known French herbalist Maurice Messegue used to prescribe an infusion of garlic, onion, savoury and mint for his patients with low libido. Hard to believe it worked, but one actor who consulted him tried it out, according to Messegue, and after a while came to see him again. 'I have a new problem,' he said. 'We can't seem to stop. Don't you have something to calm me down?'

'According to traditional Chinese medicine, impotence sometimes results from a yang deficiency, and the answer is one of the great tonic herbs. *Panax ginseng* is the most stimulating of them all. I prescribe it mainly for elderly men, with severe potency problems.'

The Chinese call ginseng the man-root, and consider it an all-round stimulant. There have been two small trials of its use in impotence, both of which came up with a success rate of around 60%. Ginseng is thought to work by dilating blood vessels, boosting blood supply to the penis and stimulating areas of the brain involved with sexual function. One snag: you may need to take ginseng for several weeks before the results show up, and genuine ginseng is expensive. Those who are on drugs for high blood pressure should not take ginseng at all (nor, by the way, should pregnant women).

For younger men, milder tonics can be just as effective. The two Peter Conway uses most are Siberian ginseng, and *Rhodiola rosea*: 'They're both effective, but I find *Rhodiola rosea* slightly has the edge on Siberian ginseng,' he says.

US herbalist Michael Tierra describes the Ayurvedic herb ashwaganda as 'almost specific for impotence'. As far as I know, there have been no good clinical trials of this effect, but what is certainly true of ashwaganda is that it can reduce anxiety, boost the immune system generally and combat physical stress, all of which might help solve a lot of performance problems.

In fact most of the reputed herbal aphrodisiacs from exotic places are valued not only for their potency-inducing powers but also as nourishing broad-spectrum tonics. The catuaba tree from northern Brazil is nicknamed 'the tree of love' and this most celebrated national aphrodisiac is also considered a great tonic for nerves, agitation and general weakness. Another famed Brazilian aphrodisiac is muira puama (*Ptychopetalum olacoide*), locally known as 'potency wood' and prized for its power to zizz up sexual performance. It's also valued as a central nervous system tonic, useful in stress and fatigue. Peruvians eat maca root like a vegetable and feed it to their livestock, but its fame as a sexual tonic is rivalled by its reputation as a terrific boost to energy and general health.

'Sex: the thing that takes up the least amount of time and causes the most amount of trouble.'
JOHN BARRYMORE, actor

Defining idea...

Poor circulation – the inability to move blood around the body efficiently – can be another factor; sufferers usually complain of cold hands and feet, and are prone to chilblains. Try wonderfully warming prickly ash, made from the bark and berries of a North American shrub, to speed things up a bit. All of these herbs are available as capsules, powders or tinctures. Buy reputable brands and follow the dosage instructions on the package.

Over lunch in a Paris bistro years ago, a handsome Frenchman whom I strongly fancied leaned over the table and told me in a low husky voice, 'Oysters are a tremendous aphrodisiac,' before ordering us a dozen each. The reason why? They're high in zinc which is crucial to male sexual performance. Fortunately there are cheaper, and year-round, sources of zinc. Pumpkin seeds are zinc rich and so are sesame seeds, which could explain why, all over the Arab world, the rich sweetmeat halvah (made from pounded sesame seeds and honey) was eaten to enhance sexual vitality and prowess. Honey itself has been credited with mild aphrodisiac powers: why else would we talk of honeymoons?

85

How did it go?

Q **I could do with a little something to gee up my performance in bed, but I can't afford any of those sexual tonics you see advertised all over the Internet. Isn't there something cheaper I could try?**

A *The answer to a man's prayer may be sitting in your kitchen cupboard. You could hardly imagine a more unlikely aphrodisiac than a bowl of porridge, but think big glossy oat-fed stallions raring to go, and eat plenty of porridge and muesli. Wild oats may be even more effective: look for the tincture and follow the dosage directions on the label. Oats may not work instant magic, but they are a wonderful all-round tonic and a great strengthener of the nervous system, which might help solve your problem another way.*

Q **I've heard that chocolate is an aphrodisiac. Sounds too good to be true – is it?**

A *Well, yes, it is a bit. Casanova, we're told, fortified himself for sex by sipping hot chocolate and we now know that chocolate contains a natural stimulant and antidepressant with a high feel-good effect. But sadly, your favourite white or milk Belgian chocolates won't do the trick. It has to be dark chocolate with at least 70% cocoa solids.*

21

Maybe baby

Failure to conceive spells misery for many couples, who wonder if their dreams will ever come true.

But even in desperate cases, IVF may not be the only answer.

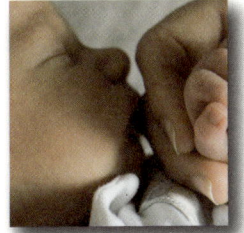

Naturopath and herbalist Francesca Naish has been treating infertile couples for more than thirty years at her clinic in Australia. Over and over again, she has proved that a comprehensive overhaul of diet, lifestyle and general health, with a continuous input of supportive herbal medicine and ongoing monitoring throughout, can have a happy outcome in the shape of a healthy bouncing baby. 'It's been suggested to me that my job description should be fairy godmother,' she laughs.

Over the years she and her carefully trained staff have successfully treated thousands of couples, many in their early forties, many with a history of miscarriage, some who have tried IVF without success, some about to try it as a last resort, and many of them diagnosed infertile. Many of them conceive within four months of starting the programme.

Couples embarking on the programme are asked to use natural contraception methods for the first four months while they get their act cleaned up. Dietary stipulations are rigorous: no coffee, alcohol or white sugar and only organic foods, to exclude pesticide and antibiotic residues. Treatment starts with a extremely

Excess pounds can diminish your chances of conception. Try *Gymnema sylvestre*, an Indian herb whose common name of gurmar actually means 'sugar destroyer'. When you take it you lose your taste for sugar, as well as the craving for sweet foods. It's sometimes combined with black pepper which contains chromium – a mineral essential to the body's metabolism of carbohydrates.

thorough detox. 'Schisandra stands out as a liver-cleanser and tonic,' Francesca says, 'and I also use dandelion, milk thistle, rosemary, lots of nettle and cleavers.'

Rosemary is a great general tonic, which improves both general digestion and liver function. It's also extremely rich in antioxidants, to protect vulnerable sperm or egg from free-radical damage. Cleavers – that odd clinging weed found in hedgerows – is another terrific cleanser, boosting lymphatic drainage to help clear wastes from the body, while milk thistle protects and stimulates the liver.

'Radiation can be a huge factor in fertility problems, affecting both DNA and chromosomes,' Francesca points out. Burdock and Siberian ginseng are two herbs she finds terrific at sorting out radiation problems; Siberian ginseng is also helpful for improving general resistance to stress, whether mental or physical.

In Francesca's programme, both men and women are treated with herbs that nourish the reproductive system and improve fertility. One outstanding herb here is *Tribulus terrestris* leaf, which has been shown to raise testosterone concentration, restore libido and up both sperm count and sperm motility. For women, she often prescribes an Indian herb, shatavari root, which in Ayurvedic medicine is considered the supreme rejuvenating tonic for women. Traditionally, shatavari is reputed to nourish and strengthen the whole reproductive system. Not for nothing, perhaps, does its Indian common name translate as 'she who possesses a hundred husbands'.

'A healthy body is a fertile body.'
FRANCESCA NAISH, herbalist

Defining idea...

Infertile couples are usually deeply stressed by months of alternating hope and despair. A great herb to know here is ashwaganda, sometimes known as Indian ginseng, and a wonderful strengthening tonic for men and women alike, which is both safe and effective. For more details of her treatment, visit www.fertility.com.au.

Even if you can't follow Francesca's programme personally, you can still learn a lot from her approach. Especially important are her insistence on the necessity of thorough cleansing and detox – using herbs such as burdock, dandelion and nettle – and the building of outstanding general health and stress resistance, calling on wonderful tonics like ashwaganda, Siberian ginseng or shatavari.

As always, however, you shouldn't take herbal medicines if you are already on prescription drugs without discussing it with your doctor. And for more specific help for complex reproductive problems, always consult a trained herbalist, who can compose your own personal prescription, matching herbs to your specific problems.

How did it go?

Q My husband and I intend to follow a detox and nutrition programme to help me conceive the baby we want so desperately. Can you tell me more about the recommended dandelion, nettles and burdock?

A *Dandelion is a bitter herb, which will help improve function throughout your digestive system, upping waste elimination through your liver and kidneys. Nettles are rich in minerals, which makes them a great tonic if you're feeling run down and low in energy. Your body needs those minerals to carry out its own ongoing detoxing, and nettles stimulate both liver and bladder. Burdock roots are another great cleansing food medicine. This useful trio are often combined in ready-made tinctures or capsules; follow the dosage instructions and give yourself at least a four-week course.*

Q My partner and I are really longing for a baby, but we've become so obsessive about it that we find it really hard to relax and enjoy sex any more. Can you help?

A *Don't try too hard, my wise mother used to say, and there are countless stories of couples who tried for months and years, then gave up and adopted – whereupon the woman immediately conceived. Forget about babies for the time being, and use a little aromatherapy to make your lovemaking the relaxing joy it should be for you both. Orange blossom was traditionally strewn around honeymoon bedrooms to relax first-night nerves: its essential oil, neroli, has the same calming anti-anxiety effect. Jasmine, with its heady, fragrance and sweet, potent ylang-ylang are other essential oils with gorgeous smells and a reputation as aphrodisiacs. Put a few drops of each in a burner in your bedroom, or add 5 drops of each to a cup of whole milk and tip into a lover's bath. Remember, essential oils should not be taken internally or applied undiluted to the skin.*

22

Time of the month

Periods don't have to be a pain.

Enlist some herbal allies to help end those monthly miseries.

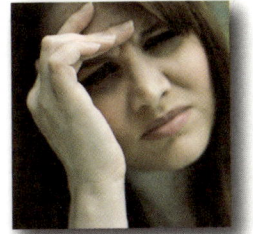

In a normal healthy woman, eating a good diet, periods should be no big deal. But if the bleed is excessive or prolonged, if it happens in between periods or if there's unusual pain in the pelvic area then or after sex, get yourself checked out by your doctor. If your GP finds nothing you should worry about, try some appropriate herbal help.

If there's one herb that really is specially for women, it has to be *Vitex agnus castus* or chasteberry, usually known just as vitex. Men have been warned off it for centuries by its reputation for suppressing their sexual urges, leaving women free to exploit its extraordinary hormone-regulating powers. Hormones out of sync are responsible for a lot of the grief in periods, and legions of modern women have learned to be thankful for vitex.

Two large surveys carried out in Germany studied its effect on 1542 women suffering from PMS over twenty-three weeks. In 90% of cases symptoms such as headache, sore breasts, mood swings, anxiety and restlessness were completely relieved. Improvement usually began within three to four weeks of starting treatment. (Don't take it, though, if you're on the contraceptive pill, HRT or if you're taking prescription drugs.)

Here's an idea for you...

When cramps are so bad that you can hardly drag yourself through the day, try something soothing. US herbalist Rosemary Gladstar suggests a hot ginger poultice. 'Make a pot of strong ginger tea by grating fresh ginger and adding it to cold water. Bring it to a low boil and simmer (with the lid tightly on) for ten to fifteen minutes. Allow it to cool just slightly. Dip a clean cotton cloth in the tea and wring out any excess liquid. Put a dry towel over the pelvic area and then place the hot poultice over it. Cover it with a thick towel, leave it on till it begins to cool, and repeat till the pain is eased.' Drink a cup of warm ginger tea sweetened with a little honey; at the same time add rosemary. That'll help ease the cramps, too.

In traditional Chinese medicine, dong quai or Chinese angelica is prescribed for almost every female complaint in the book, from menstrual cramps, irregularity and weakness through to menopausal problems. It's a warming, comforting herb, specially useful when you're feeling low and fragile. It's often combined with cramp bark – the name is self-explanatory. US herbalist Michael Tierra suggests combining equal parts of angelica, cramp bark and chamomile, plus a little grated fresh ginger root, for a calming and warming tonic for such times. Put 25g of this mix into a pan with 600ml cold water; bring it to the boil and simmer for fifteen minutes, then strain and drink hot. Dong quai should be discontinued a week before your period starts, as it may stimulate bleeding. And don't use if you are on blood-thinning drugs.

Contraceptive pills, incidentally, deplete many essential nutrients in women taking them – including zinc, magnesium, vitamins C and E and vitamin B6. Try to make up these deficiencies in your diet: eat more nuts, seeds, wholegrains, green vegetables and take a good vitamin and mineral supplement as extra insurance. If you feel your diet is inadequate, take one of the special supplements aimed at women.

The EFAs – essential fatty acids – are especially important. They are found in oily fish, and one EFA in particular, gamma-linolenic acid, or GLA, is supplied by only three to four plants, among them the lovely evening primrose, whose seeds are rich in the stuff. This EFA helps regulate hormone balance in the body, and controls the production of certain compounds called prostaglandins which may be responsible for a whole slew of PMS symptoms including mood swings, depression and – in particular – the extreme breast tenderness that some women experience. So striking is the relief it can give for this symptom that doctors in the UK are allowed to prescribe it to sufferers. Look for a good brand (the market is awash with cheap ones) and take 500mg once or twice a day.

Finally, plants that can influence human hormonal states are powerful medicine. If possible consult a herbal practitioner who can fine-tune a herbal prescription to your specific case.

'...the body normally runs its affairs very well indeed: a good medicine might therefore be one that gently nudges it back on track when it becomes disrupted.'
SIMON MILLS, author of *Woman Medicine: Vitex agnus-castus.*

Defining idea...

How did it go?

Q   **I'm really vile when my period is due – tense, irritable, emotional – and I give everyone around me a really hard time. How can I calm myself down?**

A   *You wouldn't expect a herb called passionflower to be a great sedative, but that's exactly what it is: in this case, a great calmer of hormonal mayhem. Take it in tincture form, and follow the maker's directions. It's often combined with oats, a nourishing tonic for your poor nerves, so get into the porridge habit at breakfast time.*

Q   **Help! I get really bad cramps, especially late in the evening. What can I do to ease the pain?**

A   *Try the essential oil of lavender. Smooth it into your tummy just where it hurts then add another 10–12 drops to a warm bedtime bath, which will make you feel nice and sleepy too. Another suggestion comes from German herbalists Peter and Barbara Theiss: a yarrow bath. To make it, pour a litre of boiling water over a good handful of dried yarrow and let it steep for twenty minutes, then strain and pour it into your bath. And another idea: crush 25g of caraway seeds, put them in a glass or china jug, pour 600ml of cold water over them, and leave them to steep overnight. Next morning, strain off the spicy, brown-tinged water, and take a couple of tablespoons whenever you feel your cramps coming on.*

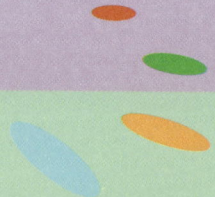

23
All change

Hot flushes, night sweats, irritability, weepiness, loss of sex drive, the blues, poor sleep – sound familiar?

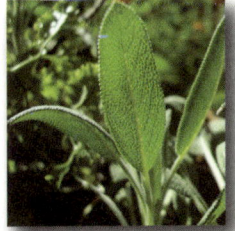

Well, of course, it's the dreaded 'change', the menopause that so many Western women are resigned to suffering.

Hormone replacement therapy or HRT once seemed to be the magical modern solution, the no-change pill that would keep us sexy, soft skinned and strong boned into ripe old age. Now women are deserting it in droves, since its long-term use has been linked with higher rates of breast cancer and stroke. And many women never got on with HRT anyway. So what's the alternative?

Try nature's own HRT: eat a diet rich in phytoestrogens, the weak hormone-like chemicals found in a huge range of foods. Think wholegrains, especially rye and oats, sesame and sunflower seeds, beans, split peas and lentils, leafy greens of all kinds, fruits, garlic, onions and soya. In cultures where diets are based mainly on such foods, breast cancer is rare and the menopause a non-event.

The natural oestrogen in your body is around a hundred times stronger than these plant hormones, but as your in-house production plummets at menopause, phytoestrogens can gently bridge the gap – usually without the problems common with HRT. There is some evidence that they can even protect us against hormone-

Here's an idea for you...

Are hot flushes and night sweats a real pain? The best remedy may be growing in your window box: common or garden sage. Make up a tea by infusing 1 tbsp of fresh sage leaves or 2 teaspoons of the dried herb in 600ml of boiling water. Let it stand, covered, for an hour and then strain it. Cool and freeze it in ice-cube trays; suck a cube several times a day.

linked cancers. In one study scientists measured the amount of phytoestrogens a group of women were eating by studying the breakdown products in their urine. They found that women with the lowest phytoestrogen count were four times more likely to develop breast cancer than the women with the highest intake.

The phytoestrogen they were testing was flaxseed oil (otherwise known as linseed oil), which is particularly rich in them, and a great food medicine. Buy a reliable blend, refrigerate immediately after opening and finish it off within two weeks. Take it by the spoonful, add it to smoothies or use it in salad dressing.

Certain herbs are especially rich in these phytoestrogens, and women the world over sussed them out among the local flora centuries ago. Around the Mediterranean, the berries of *Vitex agnus castus* or chastetree, with their heavy, powerful aroma, have been woman's medicine since Classical times. It may be especially useful during the run-up to the menopause, when the monthly cycle can become wildly erratic, with cramps, breast tenderness, headaches and occasionally heavy bleeding. *Vitex* works not by supplementing oestrogen, but by balancing hormone levels generally. Mild nausea is an occasional side effect. Don't expect it to work overnight, though; you'll need to take it for up to three months before the effect kicks in.

Russian women have used liquorice tea for centuries as a home remedy to sort out their hot flushes and help them cope with the general stress of menopause. Don't overdose on it, though, if you have a tendency to water retention – and forget it if you have high blood pressure.

'Menopause... is a beginning, not an ending; a time for looking forward, not one of sadness and regret; a time for renewal, not for a fear of ageing.'
KITTY CAMPION, *A Woman's Herbal*

Defining idea...

Asian women have their own 'female' remedy: the root of dong quai or Chinese angelica, the number one women's tonic in traditional Chinese medicine. It may not directly affect hormone levels, but it's a warmer-upper of a tonic, great for those times when menopausal women are apt to feel draggy, listless and low in energy. Beginning to think you'll never feel sexy again? Then this could be the herb for you, especially as it can help halt vaginal drying and thinning.

Phytoestrogenic herbs pack a powerful punch hormonally, and it's not a good idea to combine them with HRT or other hormonal drugs. If you decide to try them instead, consult your doctor about coming off HRT. Ideally, a professional herbalist will help work out a personal prescription for you; otherwise, try these herbs one at a time.

If loss of libido is bugging you, incidentally, copy women in the Middle East and stock up on their favourite warm-up spice, fenugreek seeds. Supposedly, the seeds are aphrodisiac; they'll also help sort out vaginal dryness, soreness and inflammation. Use them in your favourite curry or add a spoonful to a mugful of boiling water, let it stand for fifteen minutes, then strain and drink at bedtime and for breakfast.

97

How did it go?

Q   Since the menopause, my vagina often feels unbearably hot, itchy and painful. Is there a herbal remedy I can use?

A.   Herbalist Dee Atkinson gives her patients a cream containing phytoestrogen-rich wild yam and healing calendula, or suggests they insert a vitamin E capsule in the vagina two to three times a week – it dissolves and helps to repair tissue.

Q   I never normally get depressed but since my menopause started I get the blues all the time. Can you help me?

A   Try St John's wort: a whole slew of trials have demonstrated its value for states of minor depression. In one study of 111 menopausal women, symptoms such as irritability, broken sleep and depression diminished or disappeared in over 75%. As a welcome side effect, over 60% of the women reported a revived desire for sex. St John's wort should not be taken if you are on prescription drugs as it may interfere with their absorption, mind.

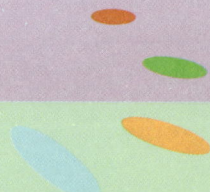

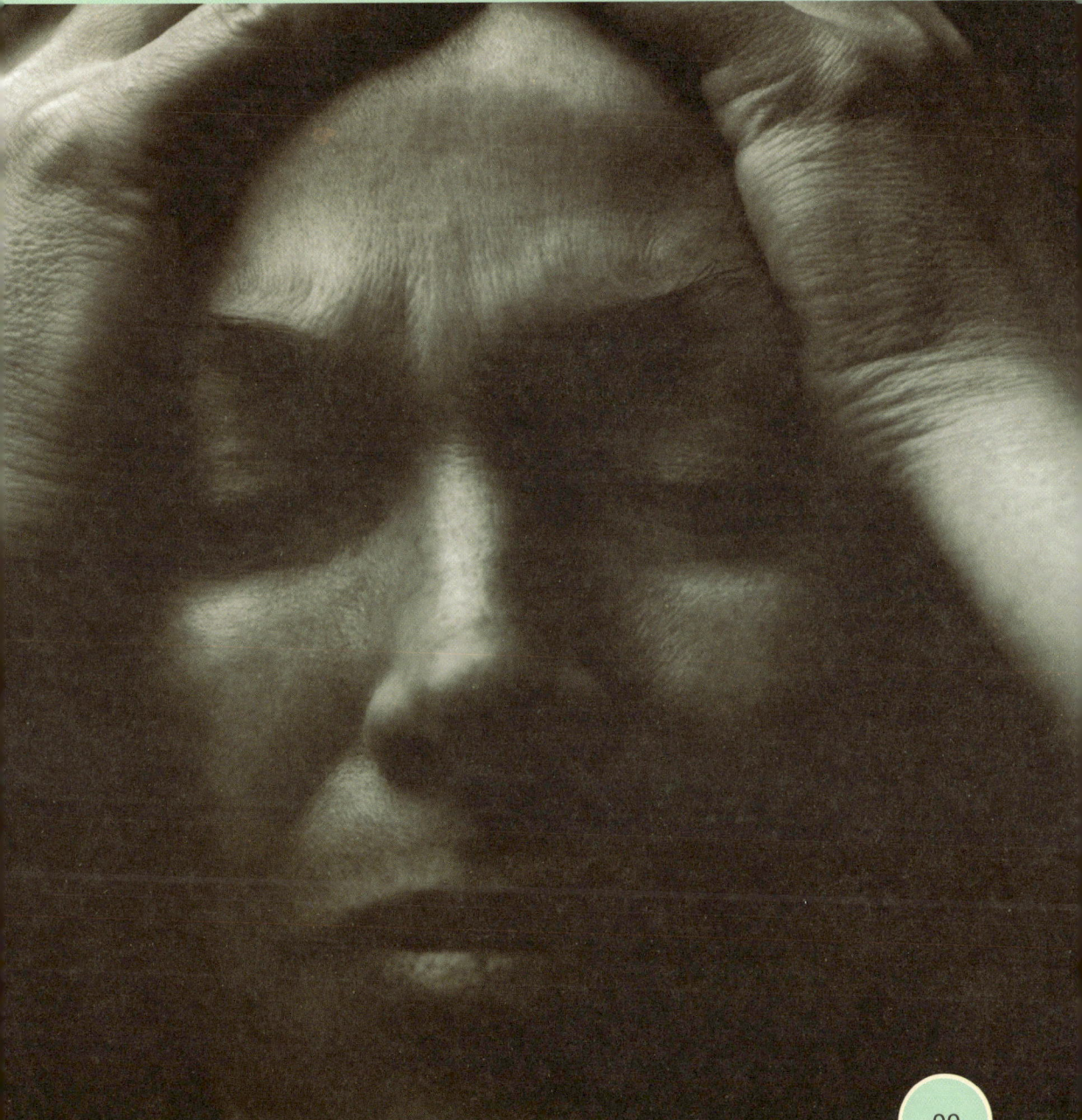

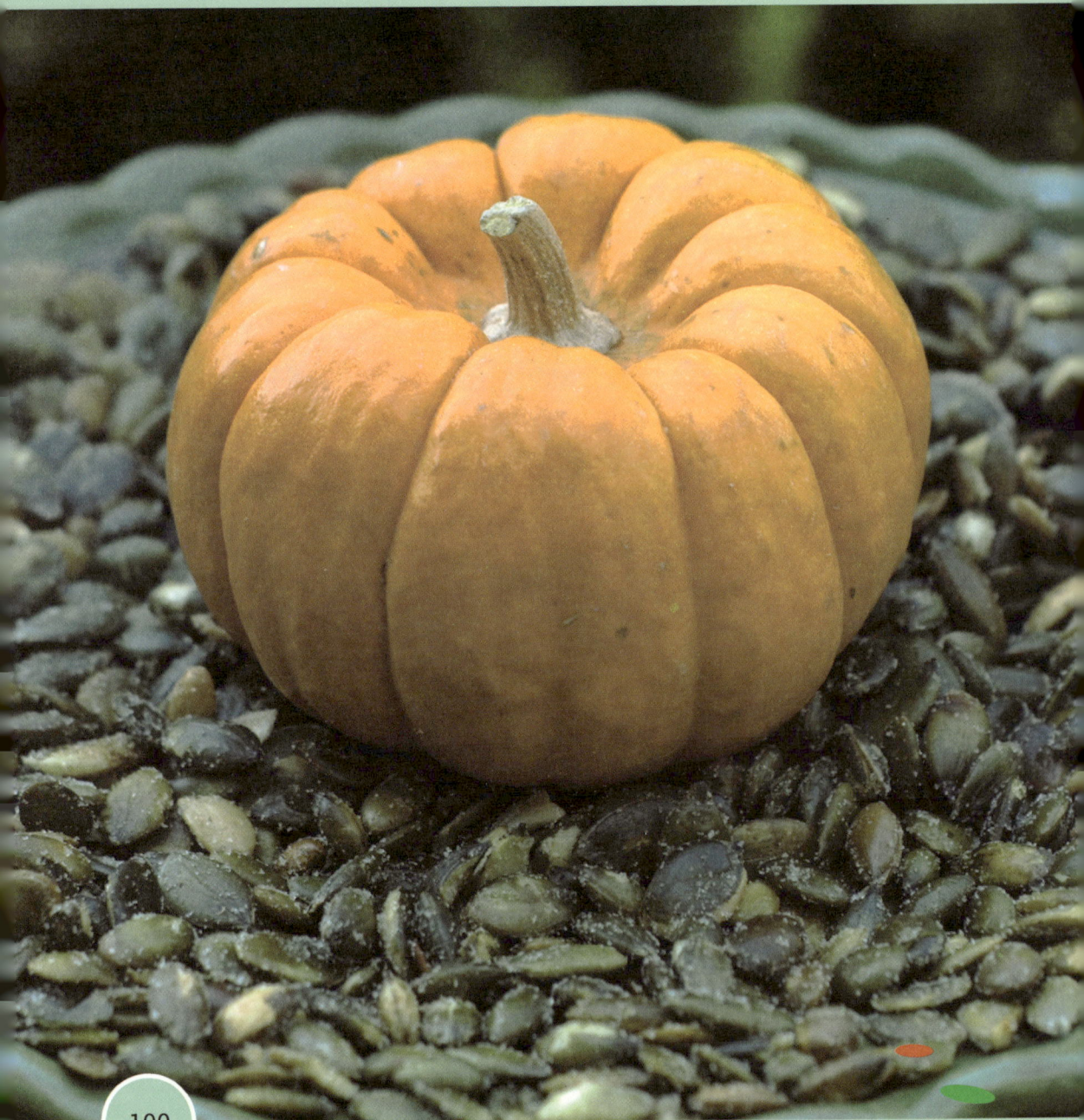

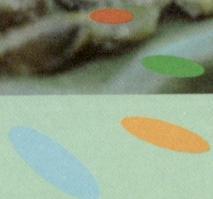

24

Male misery

If there's one word guaranteed to bring a thoughtful look to the face of any man over fifty, it's prostate.

No other part of his anatomy is more likely to give him problems.

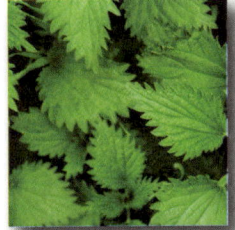

Even before the fifty-year mark, the prostate can start making its presence felt by getting infected, swollen and inflamed. This is prostatitis, which may become chronic, and your doctor will probably treat it with courses of antibiotics. Once you pass fifty, however, the gland can act up without any infectious cause. This is benign prostatic hypertrophy – BPH for short – and, like prostatitis, it's a nuisance because of its growing stranglehold on the urethra. Urine flow can slow to a trickle, and nights will more and more be broken by the urge to get up for a pee. In the long term there are more painful symptoms: a deep dull ache in the pelvic area or lower back, blood in the urine and increasing difficulty in urination.

You should see your doctor if you have any of these symptoms. However, the drugs you may be prescribed don't work for everyone and they can have disagreeable side effects, so there are excellent reasons to go for the herbal alternative. If you do decide to take any form of herbal medicine, or consult a medical herbalist, keep your doctor in the picture. It's a good idea to have a regular prostate check-up to make sure the herbs are working for you.

Here's an idea for you...

Zinc is vital for male health, especially in the prostate zone, and pumpkin seeds – those little dark green ones – are a super source. Mix a tablespoonful with a bowl of muesli: add water to cover, soak overnight, and they'll be chewy by breakfast time; or grind them and add them at once. Use pumpkin seed oil for salads, too.

The Big Three in herbal prostate treatment are saw palmetto, pygeum and nettle. Saw palmetto is an amazing little berry grown in Florida and used for centuries by the natives to alleviate men's problems; more than seventeen studies have proved its efficacy. One of these, incidentally, compared it with the standard drug treatment, finasteride, and found that it worked just as well but with fewer side effects. Several studies suggest that saw palmetto can be effective in 80 to 90% of cases. It can also be used as prevention, in courses of two to three months a year, once you've hit your fifties. Get your doctor to check you for prostate cancer before starting, as it can mask symptoms.

Pygeum africanum is an African evergreen tree that early nineteenth-century travellers found natives using for 'old man's disease'. Plenty of double-blind studies have proved its efficacy at reducing those annoying symptoms, and in France many doctors consider it the treatment of choice for BPH. It works especially well when combined with saw palmetto. However, pygeum is, sadly, on the way to the endangered list.

That's never going to be true of common-or-garden stinging nettles though, which herbalists have long prized as a useful anti-inflammatory – and a pretty nutritious herb into the bargain. At least one study has shown that it can relieve BPH symptoms, and it's often combined with saw palmetto. In spring you can add fresh young nettle tops to steamed spinach or soups. At other times you can take it in tincture form or as a tea – tea bags are available. Nettles will boost your general health; they are very rich in minerals.

Plan your prevention strategy well, though, and you may never know the misery your prostate can inflict on you, or need the dodgy drugs. And there's plenty you can do in the way of prevention.

Regular exercise is key to keeping things moving in the pelvic area. Pilates is especially good because it focuses on the often-neglected set of muscles in this area. Just walking is fine, too. Like most of the other parts of us, the prostate, too, benefits from those much-cried-up omega-3 fatty acids. Eat oily fish regularly or take linseed (otherwise known as flaxseed) in one of the many forms now available.

'I'm betting my own prostate gland that herbal treatments work better than the most commonly prescribed drugs or surgery for controlling BPH...'
DR JAMES DUKE, leading US authority on medicinal plants, *The Green Pharmacy*

Defining idea...

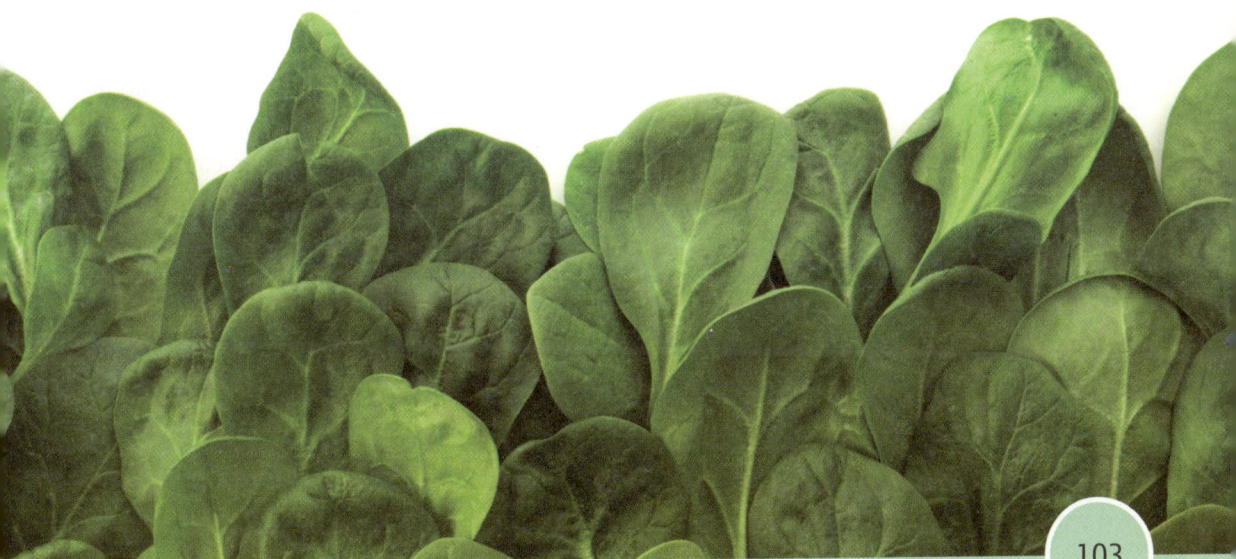

103

How did it go?

Q **I've heard that eating plenty of tomatoes can help me avoid prostate problems, and I love them anyway. How does this work?**

A *In a six-year study of prostate cancer, researchers looked at the levels of lycopene – a potent antioxidant – in the blood, and found that the risk of developing prostate cancer decreased with higher levels of lycopene. Men taking 50mg of lycopene daily had significantly higher levels in their blood. In tests for lycopene, sun-dried tomatoes in oil had the highest content. The next best source of this great stuff is processed ripe tomatoes, as found in ketchup and pasta sauces. Organically grown tomatoes, incidentally, had almost double the lycopene content of those more conventionally grown.*

Q **I've got a bad case of prostatitis and it's giving me a lot of trouble. My doctor keeps giving me antibiotics for it, but I don't want to go on taking them for too long. Any herbal suggestions?**

A *Andrographis and echinacea are both valuable boosters to your immune system, which will work well alongside the antibiotics. Two herbs, buchu and bearberry, have a specific action in the urinary tract to help clear up infections. In ready-made formulae they are often combined with marshmallow, which has a soothing effect on poor inflamed mucous membrane in the urinary tract. And make sure you eat plenty of cranberries, which have direct antibacterial action in the urinary tract. Commercial juices are high in sugar or synthetic sweeteners, but you can buy concentrated cranberry pills. Better still, buy the berries in season and freeze them to have a year-round supply: their tart taste combines well with other fruit in purées, pies, puddings.*

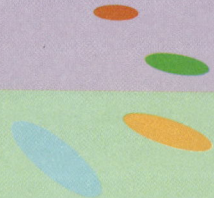

25

Winter woes

Few of us get through winter without a single cold.

But with a little herbal help you can arm yourself against infection, stop a starting cold in its tracks or, at the very least, limit the damage.

There's usually a moment when a shivery, chilly sensation warns you that a cold is on its way in. That first shiver is a sign that the viruses are already multiplying, and the battle against a cold is won or lost at this stage.

Top of any herbalist's list of great anti-cold herbs is garlic, famous in folk medicine across the planet for its protective and immune-boosting powers. It's also been more closely scrutinised by scientists than any other medicinal plant. Take the fresh cloves in heroic quantities and that cold won't stand a chance. Some friends of mine chop up and eat two or three fat fresh cloves in a thickly-buttered sandwich at the first shiver of a cold or flu – and they haven't had a cold since they started doing this some six years ago. However, lots of garlic can be an irritant to a sensitive gut, so experiment with smaller quantities first.

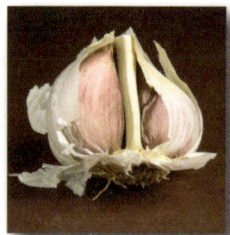

Here's an idea for you...

Onions, close cousins of garlic, share many of its wonderful healing powers. You could exploit both in this recipe sent to my husband by a friend in Angola: he swears it will see off both cold and flu bugs in short order, especially if you take it at the first suspicion of either. Peel and chop up an onion and a fat clove of garlic. Put them in a pan with the juice of a lemon, a dessertspoonful of honey and a mugful of water. Bring to the boil and simmer very slowly, covered, for forty to fifty minutes. Drink it red hot and, if you're feeling really chilled, add a spot of dried chilli powder.

Dozens of studies have demonstrated the power of echinacea to prevent, or at least diminish, the force of an oncoming cold. Once again you need to take it at the very first sign of symptoms – and in high doses. The test of a good strong echinacea is that it makes your tongue tingle a bit. If you're especially prone to colds and other bugs making the rounds in winter, consider taking echinacea in a lower dose throughout the season; it's not true, though widely believed, that you need to take regular breaks while doing so. The company founded by Swiss naturopath Dr Alfred Vogel, who pioneered the use of echinacea in Europe, makes a tincture from the fresh plants organically grown in its own gardens, as well as a chewable tablet form, handy for the desk drawer or for travel.

Elderflower is another tried and tested country remedy for colds, especially when combined with peppermint. Put a teaspoon – or a tea bag – of each in a mug, fill with hot water, strain and drink hot at an early bedtime. You'll probably sweat the cold out overnight and have a sound, sweet sleep.

For true kitchen medicine, here's a great spice-rack remedy from herbalist Dee Atkinson. Take a teaspoon each of dried sage, rosemary and thyme, put them into a teapot and add a pint of boiling water. Infuse for ten minutes, then strain and drink hot throughout the day. Another great spicy warmer-upper is ginger, which is also wonderfully stimulating: it's revered throughout the East for its many healing powers. Hot ginger tea could be your first line of defence against a threatened cold. To make it, grate a chunk of peeled, fresh ginger root into a mug, add a pinch of cardamon, fill with boiling water and infuse, covered, for ten minutes. Alternatively, add a pinch of powdered ginger to hot lemon and honey.

'A family is a unit composed not only of children, but of men, women, an occasional animal, and the common cold.'
OGDEN NASH

Defining idea...

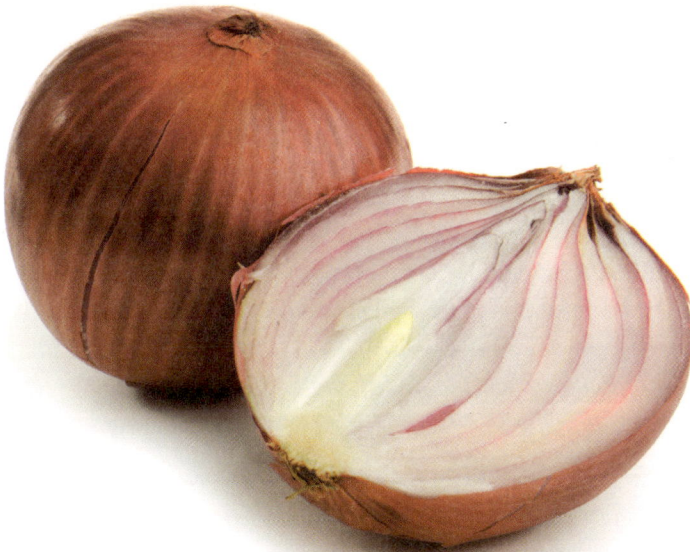

How did it go?

Q   **I've heard that the healthiest way to start the day is to drink a mug of hot water with the juice of a lemon added to it. Any comments?**

A   *It's an excellent habit. Lemon juice is cleansing, antiseptic, a fine tonic for the liver and rich in vitamin C, just the thing to protect you against a cold. But if you want to make the most of the lemon's staggering healing powers, you need to know that even more of them, especially the valuable antioxidants, are concentrated in the skin and pith. So instead of simply juicing your lemon and binning its most valuable bits, slice a whole unwaxed lemon into a mug and fill with boiling water and let it steep, covered, all night. Strain and drink the next morning – it's got a much more interesting taste, too.*

Q   **My kids are always coming down with coughs and colds. Is there a good way to nip them in the bud?**

A   *Try a mustard footbath at bedtime: it's very popular with most kids, as well. It revs up the circulation to warm them right through, and it helps check mucus build-up in the lungs. In pre-antibiotic days, a mustard plaster on the chest saved many a child stricken by whooping cough. To make the footbath, mix a heaped tablespoonful of ordinary mustard powder with hot water, stir it into a deep bowl filled with water as piping hot as young skin can stand, then get your child to sit with their feet in it for about ten minutes, topping up with more hot water from time to time, while you read them a nice bedtime story. Towel their feet dry, put them into warm socks, and then straight into bed. Sweet dreams...*

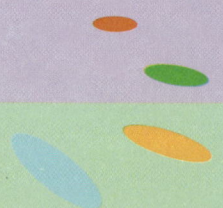

26

Rasping in the rib cage

Who needs bronchitis – the fever, the exhausting cold, the general lassitude?

Nip it in the bud with antiseptic herbs and warming spices.

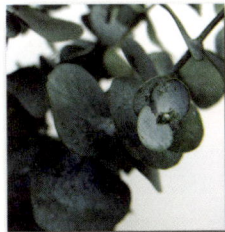

If you're prone to bronchitis, zap any respiratory infection promptly with high-dose echinacea or propolis. Keep your neck and chest warm: wear a silk or woollen scarf outdoors. Rediscover vests and sleep with your bedroom window closed on cold nights. Be lavish with warming spices – cinnamon, cloves, cardamom, and especially cayenne, which thins mucus. Eat plenty of infection-fighting garlic, onions, turnips and watercress. Cut right back on mucus-producing dairy foods – milk, butter and cheese.

If your bronchitis regularly drags on through most of winter, you've got the chronic kind – and if you are a smoker, this shouldn't surprise you. Constant irritation of the bronchii by tobacco smoke, fog or airborne pollutants of one kind or another will keep your lungs clogged with mucus.

Don't battle on with active bronchitis as you could end up with pneumonia (and spread your bugs around, too). Stay in bed and drink plenty of hot herbal teas, including peppermint and elderflower. One of the best drinks is home-made lemonade. Slice whole well-scrubbed lemons into a jug, pour boiling water over

Here's an idea for you...

Garlic is the king of plant antibiotics. Here's a delicious way to take it, suggested by famous French aromatherapist Dr Jean Valnet; if you're inclined to be chesty, make this at the start of winter. Peel and bruise 4–5 fine fresh garlic cloves, put them in a jar with an airtight screw top and add 50ml of alcohol (vodka is fine). Close the jar and leave it to macerate for three weeks. Take 20–30 drops two to three times a day. If you want to avoid alcohol, add the drops to a cup of boiling water; the alcohol will evaporate off.

them, add a little brown sugar or honey and let the mixture stand for two to three hours or overnight. Lemons – especially their rinds – are packed with compounds to boost resistance and help you fight infection.

There are lots of herbs which have been prized down the centuries for their efficacy in problems for your poor susceptible lungs. Lay in a stock of some of them from a herbal supplier and get brewing! Here are some ideas.

If the coughing is hard and sore, use the grey woolly leaves of the tall golden-flowered mullein, a soothing and anti-inflammatory expectorant and a prized traditional remedy. Infuse 1–2 teaspoons of the dried leaves in a mug filled with boiling water, and strain through coffee filter paper to get rid of all those tiny hairs. Drink it three times a day.

To calm that irritating cough, here's a useful combination: dried horehound herb and marshmallow leaves. Mix and put a good teaspoonful in a mugful of boiling water in which you have already simmered a stick of liquorice, very soothing to the throat. Infuse for ten minutes, strain and drink.

The leaves of the eucalyptus tree contain an essential oil which is strongly antiseptic. Eucalyptus oil not only helps see off bacterial and viral infections, but also soothes irritated mucous membranes and helps expel mucus. You can use dried eucalyptus leaves to make a tea effective for both acute and chronic bronchitis. Put 3–4 dried leaves in a pan, add a cupful of cold water, bring to the boil and simmer for a minute, then take off the heat, cover and let it steep for ten minutes. Strain, add a little honey and drink hot two to three times a day.

Steaming helps loosen mucus in the lungs; add some antiseptic essential oils to the mix. Put 2 drops of eucalyptus, 1 each of pine and thyme and 1 drop of lavender in a big bowl of boiling water. Let it cool just a little and then, using a towel round your head and the bowl, inhale for two to three minutes. Do this twice a day.

'The antiseptic properties of aromatic essences are put to good use every day by the housewife who uses garlic, thyme, lemon, cloves and other spices in her kitchen.'
DR JEAN VALNET, in *The Practice of Aromatherapy*

Defining idea...

How did it go?

Q   I've got a flourishing thyme plant in my garden: I know it's good for colds and bronchitis. What's the best way to use it?

A   *Drink lots of thyme tea in the winter when you have a heavy chesty cold or bronchitis; it's particularly good for people with chronic bronchitis. Add a good sprig to a mug, fill it with boiling water and steep, covered, for ten minutes. Strain and drink it hot two to three times a day. Thyme thins all that lung-clogging phlegm and helps you cough it up. It's also a terrific tonic to the immune system and has noted antiseptic powers – just what the doctor ordered. Dr Valnet suggests taking a thyme bath: put a big bunch into a large pan with 4 litres of water, bring to the boil and simmer for ten minutes, covered. Then strain it and add the water to a warm bedtime bath.*

Q   I'm very susceptible to bronchitis in the winter, and I get worn out by the coughing. Have you any ideas?

A   *Try hot ginger tea. US herbalist Stephen Harrod Buhner points out in his book* Herbal Antibiotics *that ginger's anti-cough action rivals that of codeine. It will help thin all that clogging mucus, and move it up and out of the body. 'Ginger,' he adds, 'relieves pain, stimulates immune activity, reduces inflammation and stimulates sweating, thus helping lower fevers.' To make a tea, grate an inch of peeled fresh root ginger into a mug, fill it with boiling water, and infuse, covered, for ten minutes. Strain, add a little honey, and drink hot.*

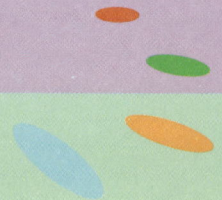

27

Throaty

Sore throats can be a painful side effect of colds or bronchitis.

But don't rush to your doctor for antibiotics: there are plenty of potent antiseptics in the plant world which will see off both viral or bacterial bugs.

Get professional help, though, if the sore throat is severe, lasts more than four or five days, or keeps coming back.

France's Dr Jean Valnet, who was a great believer in country cures, was enthusiastic about the powers of blackberry leaves to sort out a bad sore throat. Most people can locate that invasive pest the sharp-thorned bramble somewhere near them, if not in their own back garden. Arm yourself with stout gardening gloves, harvest a bagful of the prickly leaves and get to work. Put a good handful of leaves in a pan, cover with a litre of water, bring to the boil and simmer for two minutes. Then let them steep for another ten minutes. Strain through coffee filter paper – it's very important to get rid of all those tiny prickles – then drink hot three times a day. From time to time, gargle with the mix as well.

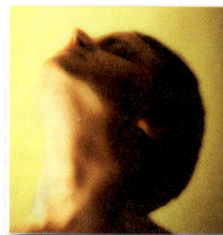

Here's an idea for you... **Try some liquorice tea to soothe that painfully inflamed and aching throat. Put three or four liquorice root sticks in a pan and cover with water. Bring to the boil and simmer for twenty minutes, then strain and enjoy. By the way, this has to be the brownish root – that popular black confectionery won't do the trick.**

Blackberry leaves, incidentally, were often used as a substitute for ordinary tea in the days when it was an expensive luxury. They have an aromatic, slightly smoky taste not unlike China tea.

Purple – or even ordinary – sage is another great country cure for sore throats: put 2 tablespoons of the fresh leaves into a pint of cold water, bring it to the boil, then leave it to steep, covered, for ten minutes. Then strain and gargle with it, two to three times a day and again at bedtime, warming it up each time. If you can't get hold of fresh sage, use a teaspoon of the dried version from your herb rack, as long as it's still fresh enough to have a good strong smell. Even better, combine the sage tea with equal parts of apple cider vinegar. You can put this mixture into a little spray bottle from the chemist and spray your throat at intervals, too.

I once recommended sage for sore throats in a newspaper article. I had a letter from a reader a week later saying that she had been having antibiotic treatment for her chronic laryngitis for over six months. On reading my suggestion she had rushed into her garden, picked a bunch and started dosing herself with sage tea. Her laryngitis had cleared in days.

Propolis, the sticky resin that bees manufacture from various tree buds for the construction of their hives, is highly antiseptic, particularly for the mouth or throat, and I've seen it work for many friends to whom I've suggested it. Add 10–20 drops to a little warm water, which will turn a cloudy yellow. Then gargle with the water, keeping the liquid in contact with your throat as long as possible; swallow it afterwards. Repeat two to three times a day.

'A good listener is not someone with nothing to say. A good listener is a good talker with a sore throat.'
KATHERINE WHITEHORN, British author and journalist

Defining idea...

Another powerful resin is myrrh, extracted from a small shrubby North African tree, and prized by ancient civilisations as perfume, incense or medicine. Tincture of myrrh is a great healer and antiseptic: add a teaspoonful to a small glass of warm water and gargle with it. *Don't* swallow this one afterwards – but it's so bitter tasting that you won't be tempted.

In Indian traditional medicine turmeric is a popular remedy for sore throats. It is in fact pain-relieving, anti-inflammatory and antiseptic. If you want to try the turmeric treatment add half a teaspoon of turmeric powder and half a teaspoon of salt to a small cup of hot water, stir well, and gargle with it. One thing: those pretty little jars of spices often hang around the kitchen for years, losing both flavour and medical usefulness. Make sure your turmeric is still fresh, bright and strongly scented.

How did it go?

A   *This painful complication of tonsillitis, an abscess at the back of one tonsil, is mercifully rare these days. If you develop the symptoms – fever, swelling in the neck glands, increasing difficulty in swallowing or even opening your mouth – get professional help fast. In the days when medical help was hard to come by, there was a popular country remedy for quinsy: a soothing, cooling, anti-inflammatory jelly made from the quinsy berry, as the blackcurrant was once called. Spectacularly high in vitamin C, the jelly was taken in teaspoon doses three or four times a day; a remedy that any child can be easily persuaded to take. Blackcurrant bushes grew wild all over Britain, and if it was too early for the fruits, a tea was made from the leaves and used as a gargle.*

Q   **Every time I get a cold I lose my voice. Can you suggest a solution?**

A   *Bill Clinton's hoarseness was often obvious to his audience. On the campaign trail, according to reports, he relied on a throat-coating tea which soothed his throat enough to let him carry on speaking. Many professional singers follow his example. Key ingredients in the tea? Herbs rich in mucilage that provide a protective coating to inflamed or irritated mucous membranes, among them liquorice root and slippery elm bark. French actors swear by cabbage juice – especially from the dark red variety of cabbage – with a little honey added to it. They use it as a gargle, then swallow it.*

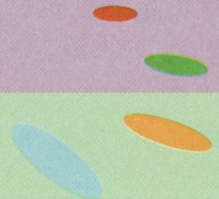

28

A bad wheeze

If you're one of the growing millions of asthmatics, life is a struggle.

You can make it a lot easier if you add a handful of helpful herbs to your coping strategies.

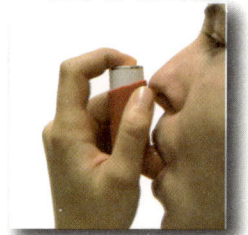

Today's rocketing figures for asthma may be due to the ever-increasing numbers of polluting chemicals in our homes. Top of the suspects in a study published in the journal *Thorax* were disinfectant, bleach, aerosols and air fresheners. And don't forget the thousands more in processed foods, drinks, toiletries, laundry products, cosmetics and perfumes. Asthma can also be caused by food sensitivities, so keep a diet diary to help you match certain foods or drinks to asthmatic episodes. Before you explore any other form of self-help, go green in your home, your kitchen and at table. Then see what herbs can do for you. If possible, consult a professional herbalist, who will work to help you reduce your dependence on your ventilator.

The following herbs work to relax constricted airways, and help your lungs expel all that clogging mucus: grindelia, coltsfoot, mullein, marshmallow, thyme and hyssop. Make up a tea from one or more of these, dried – a teaspoon infused for ten minutes in a cup of boiling water – and drink it regularly.

Here's an idea for you...

If wheezing makes it hard to get to sleep, or wakes you up during the night, try a bedtime chest rub. Add 10 drops of lavender oil to a tablespoonful of almond or olive oil, and stroke it into your chest. Lavender is a muscle relaxant so your airways won't seize up while you're sleeping, and it's so calming it will help you sleep.

A viral respiratory infection often signals the first onset of asthma, and any subsequent infection will make it much worse. Keep your immune defences in place. One of the best immunity-boosting herbs is echinacea: look for a quality product, and take courses of it at cold, damp times of the year when you are most susceptible. Ashwaganda is another great calming tonic; take a course of it before winter.

Elderflower is useful for fighting off infections, too. Use a good teaspoon of the dried flowers to a cupful of boiling water, infused for five to ten minutes, then drunk two to three times a day, the last time in bed at night. Elderberries have antiviral clout: in one study, an extract of elderberry helped subjects see off the flu virus fast – 90% within two to three days. Keep a bottle handy and start taking it at the first shiver of a cold or flu.

Around 75% of childhood asthma, and up to 20% of adult cases, are allergy related. Did you know that the common nettle is one of the most effective antihistamines around? When they're young and fresh, add nettle leaves to soups or steam them with other greens. Later in the year, drink nettle tea: it tastes a bit bland and boring, so liven it up with a little peppermint, which will help thin the mucus in your lungs. If you're seriously bored by herbal teas, order a nettle tincture from a reliable supplier and follow the dosage directions they suggest.

Inhale an essential oil and it goes straight to your lungs: even applied to your skin, it will be excreted via your lungs. So essential oils can be key players in the asthma field, and a lovely soothing massage by a trained aromatherapist could be a very therapeutic treat. Three especially helpful oils are benzoin, which is warming, antiseptic and helps thin and expel mucus; frankincense, which deepens and slows the breathing to calm you down; and tranquillising, relaxing lavender. Pine and thyme are other great choices for lung problems. It's not advisable to use them in a steam inhalation as the heat may make matters worse, but you can use them in a burner next to your desk or your favourite armchair, or inhale them from a hanky.

Asthma doesn't seem to bother me any more unless I'm around cigars or dogs. The thing that would bother me most would be a dog smoking a cigar.
STEVE ALLEN

Defining idea...

The French aromatherapist Dr Jean Valnet formulated a special mix of lung-friendly oils including pine, thyme, rosemary and lavender; you can spray this around your bed to help keep night-time wheezes at bay, use it in a burner beside your desk, or simply inhale it three to four times a day from a hanky.

To be asthmatic is to be stressed, and oats can help break the vicious cycle of stress triggering attacks which in turn pile on more stress. A tincture of the fresh whole green oat plant has helped numbers of people come off tranquillisers – a notoriously tough addiction to break. Oats are often combined with passionflower, another great calmer of fraught nerves. Hops, lemon balm, chamomile, skullcap, limeflowers and valerian are other mood-lifting, relaxing or sedative herbs, and health-food stores will have a wide range of these, singly or in combination, to choose from. Or drink them as simple teas.

How did it go?

Q **I've heard that asthmatics should eat a lot of garlic. Why is this supposed to be helpful?**

A *Garlic works two ways to help you, so eat plenty of it, preferably raw. It's very rich in a plant chemical called quercetin that damps down the inflammation that constricts your airways. And it's a powerful antimicrobial that helps fight infection: bacteria flourish in accumulated mucus. Onions share these useful qualities to a lesser degree. Use both in a delicious soup: cut up a large onion, and simmer in a little chicken broth till it's soft. When you're ready to eat it, add a lump of butter, a big clove of garlic, crushed, and a dash of cayenne pepper. Don't overdose on garlic if you're on blood-thinning drugs, aspirin or facing surgery within the next week.*

Q **I'm asthmatic and somebody told me I shouldn't be drinking tea. Is this right?**

A *Well, no. Ordinary tea is actually recommended for asthmatics, because it contains high levels of theophylline, stuff that helps open up constricted airways. Green tea likewise, and it's richer in antioxidants. Sadly, though, if you want to get the benefit of either, you'll need to drink it without milk. Some people find this very hard. Try experimenting with different teas, or add a little lemon and sugar. Or enjoy Morocco's national cuppa: green tea with sugar and a bunch of fresh mint.*

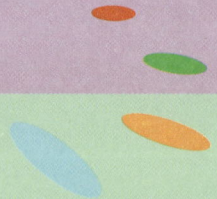

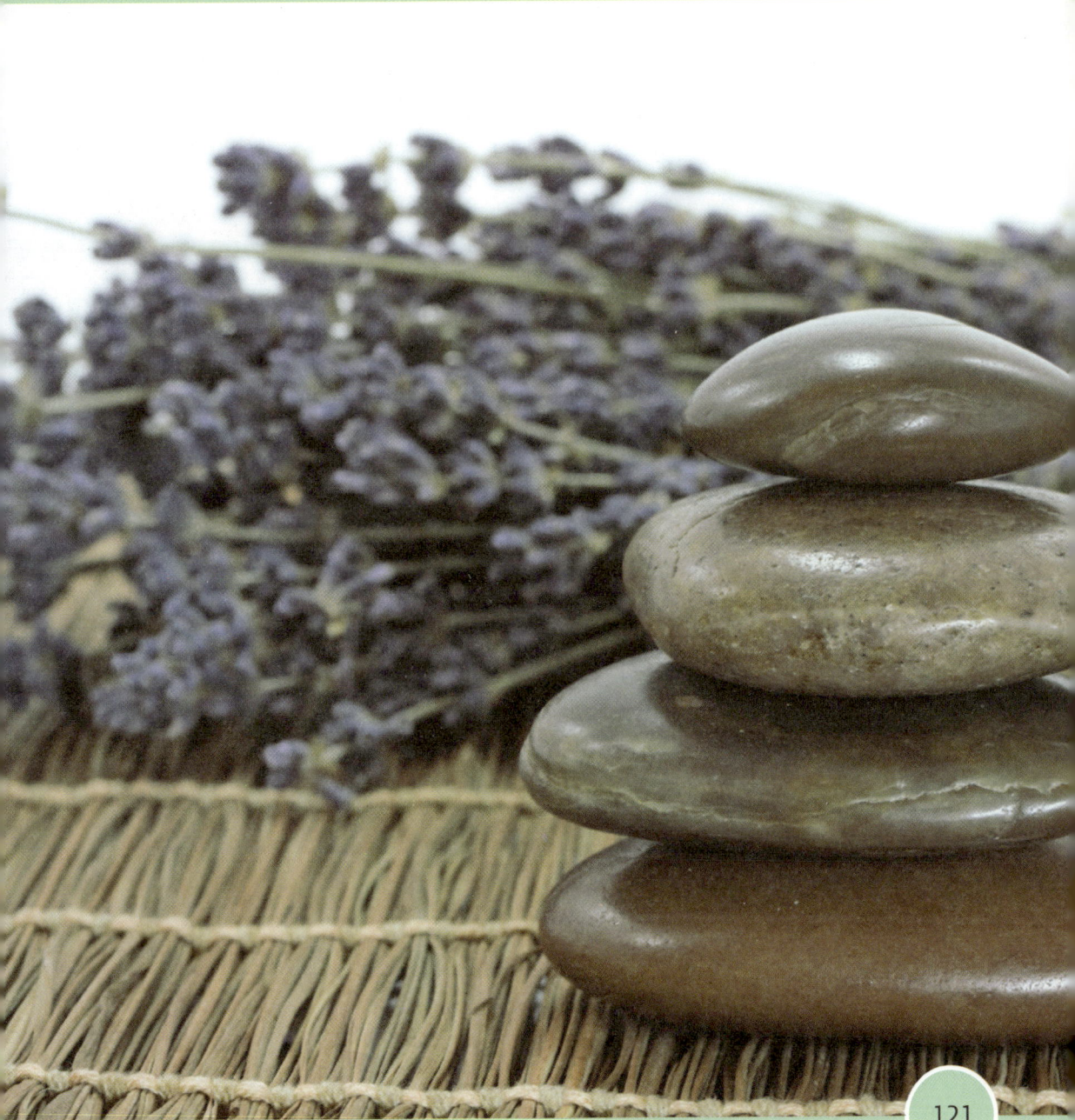

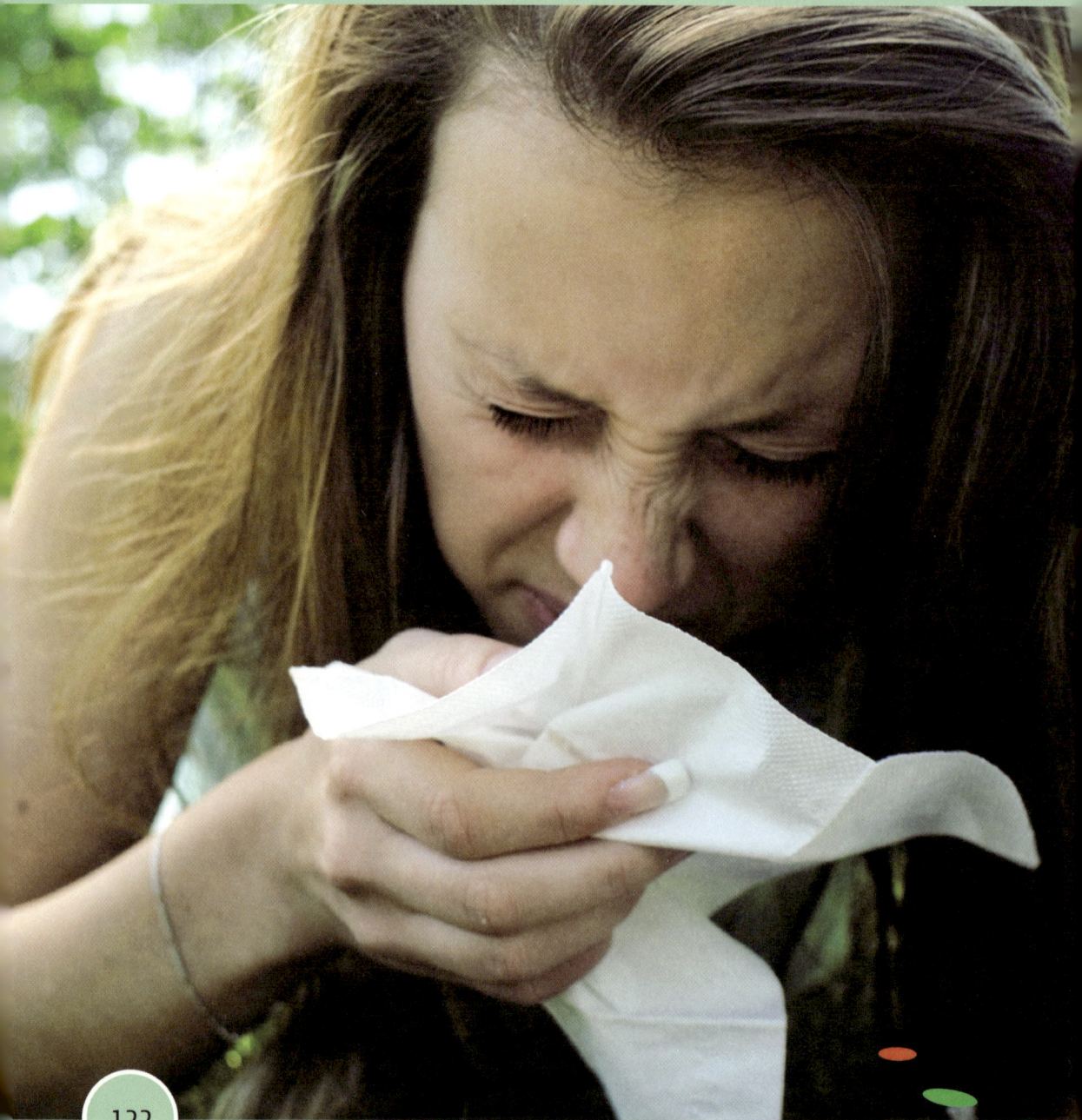

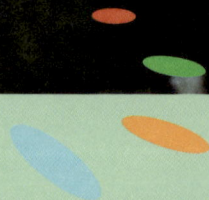

29

Atishoo!!

For millions of unhappy people, summer is the start of the hay-fever season and the big sneeze.

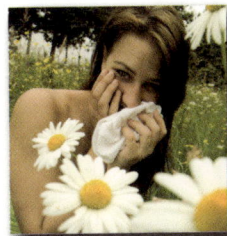

If you're one of them, use herbs to pacify the discomfort, the streaming eyes and nose, and the irritation of this condition.

Hay fever is an overreaction of our immune systems. When tree or grass pollens come in contact with the mucous membranes of eyes, nose, throat or lungs, they can trigger an allergic response to prompt the release of histamine and other inflammatory chemicals from tissue cells. Hence the wheezing, sneezing and the maddening itch around eyes and nose – which in turn produce the fatigue, the inability to concentrate and the irritability which sufferers struggle vainly to control.

Most sufferers find that the antihistamine pills which they rely on to get them through cause few side effects other than drowsiness, but that what works one season often fails the next. Try the herbal alternatives.

Top of the list are the creamy flowers of the elder tree, which in some countries are in full bloom in country hedgerows just as the hay-fever season hits its peak. Put three or four of the well-washed fresh flower heads in a glass or china teapot, pour a litre of boiling water over them and infuse for five minutes, then strain. Keep the

Here's an idea for you...

If the streaming, itchy, irritated eyes of hay fever are driving you to distraction, keep a bottle of distilled witch hazel in your fridge. From time to time soak cotton-wool pads in this soothing, icy liquid, and use them as eye compresses for ten minutes. Cooled chamomile or elderflower tea bags will work well too.

liquid warm with a tea cosy and drink three cups a day. You can buy ready-made elderflower teabags or an elderflower cordial which is, in effect, a concentrated syrup. Diluted with water, apple juice or white wine, it's a delicious summer drink in its own right. Something to celebrate? Elderflower 'champagne'.

The common stinging nettle offers wonderful relief for hay-fever symptoms. In a double-blind randomised study, 98 sufferers took 300mg of freeze-dried nettle three times a day for a week. Of these, 68% rated it moderately or highly effective, while 48% also found it as good as, or better than, the antihistamine medication they had been taking.

When my Dutch husband – a long-term hay-fever sufferer – went to his Amsterdam gym one summer morning, he spotted an interesting suggestion on the notice board. A fellow member had found that a Chinese herb called *Scutellaria baicalensis* had been extremely effective for his own severe hay fever; he urged fellow-sufferers to give it a go. Curious, my husband tried it as recommended, with a gram of vitamin C and some vitamin E. He found it worked even better than his favourite antihistamine. Word has got around in Holland, and most health-food shops in Amsterdam lay in stocks of *scutellaria* root capsules come summer. Almost certainly, it owes its new Western reputation to well-known Australian herbalist Kerry Bone, who studied Chinese and Japanese research on this traditional Chinese remedy, noted that it seemed to have striking antiallergic and anti-inflammatory effects, and began prescribing it for his hay-fever patients. He found it to be very successful, mentioned it in his book *Chinese and Ayurvedic Herbal Medicine*, and the word spread. The root, Kerry points out, is very rich in flavonoids which actually inhibit the release of histamine by cells.

Dioscorides, the author of the first Western herbal and a surgeon with the Roman armies, used eyebright to treat his soldiers' eye infections. Valued for centuries as a sovereign remedy for the eyes, it helps clear accumulated mucus, reduces the irritable sensitivity of tissue in the nose and sinuses, and calms inflammation in and around the eyes. It also strengthens oversensitive mucous membrane. Modern herbalists prescribe it to help relieve the burning, itchy eyes of hay fever. Take it in pill form or as a tincture.

If you're a hay-fever victim, your immune system is badly in need of a boost. Start a course of echinacea well before the season kicks in. The omega-3 essential fatty acids in linseed help subdue the inflammation which produces the streaming eyes and nose and the general irritation of hay fever. Take a tablespoonful of the oil every day, or grind a tablespoonful of the fresh golden seed into your morning porridge or muesli. Eat plenty of apples, berries and red or yellow onions too: they're rich in a flavonoid called quercetin which helps quell inflammation.

Defining idea…

'Human beings entirely depend on plant life to sustain us: not only are plants the source of all our food, but they create the air we breathe and are the source of all our medicines'
SUSAN CURTIS, ROMY FRASER and IRENE KOHLER, in *Neal's Yard Natural Remedies*

125

How did it go?

Q **Please help me – isn't there some sort of barrier I can put between my poor nose and those wretched pollens?**

A *Hoods, masks, helmets, nosebags packed with cotton wool, they've all been tried. But a cream claiming to be just the very barrier you're looking for was voted best organic product at the UK Natural Trade Show of 2006. It's a blend of beeswax and organic vegetable oils which you stroke on just inside your nostrils, to provide a physical barrier to pollen entry. It comes either plain, or with a touch of either frankincense or lavender essential oils – either of which may enhance its effect.*

Q **I've heard that honey can help my hay fever. Does it really work?**

A *In 1937 Captain Dr George McGrew, a military surgeon in the US Army, quizzed a number of hay-fever sufferers among his men on the home remedies that had worked for them. He reported in a medical journal that 'one alone seemed of real value... the eating of honey produced in their vicinity and particularly from the chewing of the comb wax'. In fact this treatment was a long-established traditional remedy: take a teaspoonful of honey or chew a teaspoonful of honeycomb three times a day, starting at least four months before the start of the season. The honey should be pure, unprocessed and unheated; try your local farmers' market. Why does the honey treatment work? The jury is still out, but the plant pollens in honey are rich in anti-inflammatory bioflavonoids and there are reports of the successful use of honey as a treatment for asthma.*

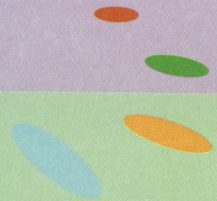

30

Nose block

Your nose is stuffed up, with a running leak to it, your mouth is dry and there's a steady dull ache around the bridge of your nose.

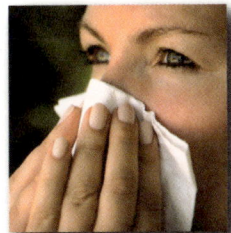

Yes, it's those wretched sinuses again. Try some herbal de-blocking.

You've got four pairs of sinuses. They're tiny air-filled cavities, clustered in the bones around your nose, and they're vulnerable to infection from viruses, bacteria, fungi, whatever. Once they've picked up any infection, that moist mucous lining becomes irritated, swollen and inflamed, producing a steady drip of mucus. As the mucus thickens and builds up, it eventually blocks your sinuses, producing that familiar bunged-up feeling as well as a dull ache.

Most cases of sinusitis develop during a cold or chest infection, and clear soon after. But they can linger on, and in many people they become chronic, resistant to any amount of antibiotic or decongestant treatment. You may find that cutting out dairy products produces dramatic relief: worth trying for a week. Chronic sinusitis can cause repeated chest infections from the steady drip of infected mucus down the air passages. If the problem persists or becomes very painful, see your doctor.

But it's well worth trying natural herbal remedies first – and there are herbs that can help you deal with both acute and chronic kinds.

Here's an idea for you...

Steaming reaches the parts other herbs may not – especially if you add one or two of the half-dozen essential oils which are good at relieving congestion and combating infection – eucalyptus, peppermint, lavender and tea tree are all good choices. Add 3–4 drops of one of these oils (or a mix) to a bowl of steaming water. Let it cool a little if it has just come off the boil so that you don't scald yourself and then tent your head and the bowl in a towel. Breathe in the aromatic steam for five minutes. Do this night and morning for a week. Do be careful: essential oils should never be taken internally, and keep them out of children's reach.

If simple remedies don't work, a qualified herbalist could help sort out the various factors giving you that permanently blocked nose – with digestive problems high on the list – and then use herbs to dry out mucus, clear blocked sinuses, and repair damage to the inflamed and irritated mucous membrane. Among the herbs they might call on are eyebright, which works locally to calm inflammation, plantain to help stem mucus output and reduce swelling, yarrow for its antiseptic and anti-inflammatory action and calendula to stimulate your resistance to infection.

If the first winter cold sees your sinusitis starting up again, take preventive action: a course of echinacea, the wonder herb that helps boost your resistance. You can take it in a low dose throughout the winter months, then switch to a higher dose, taken several times a day, at the first hint of trouble.

Two great infection-busters are propolis and garlic. Propolis is made by bees working on resins gathered from specific plants: they plaster this sticky stuff all over their hives to keep out infections, and it is especially useful for the nose, mouth and throat area. You can buy propolis combined with echinacea in tablet form, and you can also use a few drops of the sticky tincture in a little warm water as a regular gargle.

Garlic has been renowned since antiquity as an infection-fighter – it was brought to Britain by the surgeons of Roman legions posted from sunny Italy to damper, colder northern

'The patient with sinusitis has a head full of rubbish..'
ROBYN KIRBY, *Herbs for Healing*

Defining idea...

climates. Compounds in raw garlic have antibiotic action but some of garlic's efficacy – though not all – is lost in cooking. So eat plenty of raw garlic chopped in salads, or a clove crushed into soup at the last minute. To fight acute infections, take garlic in pill form and high doses – but do remember that it can irritate your stomach.

Elderflowers, like the berries, have mild antiviral action. Drink plenty of elderflower tea; use a tea bag or a teaspoonful of the dried flower heads infused for five minutes in a cupful of boiling water. It's one of the nicest of herbal infusions – drink it hot at bedtime with a little honey.

Horseradish is an age-old remedy for colds and sinus infections and now we know why. Studies carried out at the California University School of Medicine, quoted in Jean Carper's great book *The Food Pharmacy*, demonstrated that horseradish, like many other spicy foods, triggers a flash flood of fluid in air passages which thins congested mucus so that it is easily expelled; hence the watering eyes. In his lovely collection of herbal remedies, *The Green Pharmacy*, US herbal authority James Duke suggests making up a 'Sinusoup': 'Begin with your vegetable minestrone and add heaped helpings of garlic and onions, plus horseradish, hot pepper and ginger. On a cold winter day, it warms the soul as it opens the sinuses.'

How did it go?

Q **I get bored with peppermint and chamomile. Can you suggest a nice spicy tea for winter?**

A *Fenugreek makes a delicious spicy tea, which helps clear excess mucus from the respiratory system. Crush a teaspoon of the seeds and simmer them, covered, in a cupful of water for five minutes.*

Q **I'd love an instant cure for sinusitis. Does it exist?**

A *I don't know about instant, but try this wonderful aromatic sniffer. French aromatherapist Dr Jean Valnet combined a number of essential oils that work exceptionally well on the respiratory system – lavender, niaouli (Melaleuca viridiflora, related to tea tree), Scotch pine, peppermint and thyme – in a blend that he christened Climarome and packaged in atomiser bottles. For congested sinuses, he suggested spraying two to three bursts into a pocket handkerchief, then inhaling the marvellous pine-forest smells from it for a couple of minutes four times a day. For extra effect, spray it all around your pillow and bedding just before you go to bed.*

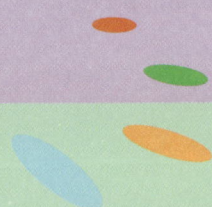

31

Knotty problems...

Varicose veins are not only unsightly but also a signal of serious damage.

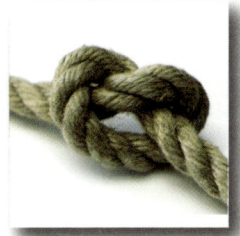

Varicose veins and piles are aspects of the same problem: veins that have become weakened and distended with blood, which can no longer efficiently perform their job of returning blood to the heart.

The circulating blood in your body relies on muscles pumping in your legs and pelvic floor to push it back up to the heart again through a series of small valves. If these muscles spend too many hours idle, blood flow slows, the valves weaken and blood begins to pool in the veins, straining and weakening their walls, and eventually leaking into surrounding tissue. That produces those typical unsightly knots, bulges and skeins of purplish thread veins. Once circulation is seriously impaired, you're at risk of hard-to-heal varicose ulcers and of deep vein thrombosis.

Varicose veins run in some families. You're at risk, too, if you spend a lot of your working life either standing or sitting around, if you're on the heavy side or if you smoke. And if you eat mainly highly refined and processed foods – white flour, sugar, cakes, pies, biscuits, etc – you've got them coming to you. Constipation is also

Here's an idea for you... **The distilled extract of witch hazel is marvellous stuff: it cools, calms inflammation and contains 'vitamin P' – bioflavonoids – to protect capillaries and small veins. Keep a big bottle of it in your fridge, and apply it to varicose veins at the end of long, tiring days. Add a little witch hazel to marigold tea and it will be even more effective when you use it to bathe your legs. An ice-cold swab of witch hazel is helpful for piles, too.**

a major risk factor. Switch to a healthier menu of vegetables, fruits, wholegrains and legumes. If your varicose veins are a really bad case, you need to see a doctor. Get them sorted before they get that serious.

Regular brisk exercise and plenty of fibre in your diet will go far to minimising damage. Treat your legs to regular cold showers. Eat plenty of leeks, garlic, onions, oats and carrots, all excellent for the circulation, as are warming spices like ginger, cinnamon and cayenne.

A quintet of herbs are especially useful in cases of varicose veins: horse chestnut, butcher's broom, *Ginkgo biloba*, gotu kola and marigold. Horse chestnuts, those glossy brown conkers that schoolchildren love, have for centuries been a popular European folk remedy for circulation problems. Their efficacy has been confirmed in a number of studies, which have shown that horse chestnut not only reduces pain and swelling, but actually works to tone and strengthen the veins, so that blood flow gradually improves. Horse chestnut can be toxic in overdose, so choose your brand carefully, and follow the directions on the label. It's also available as a gel that you can stroke gently upwards into your legs every day for a local boost to the circulation. Butcher's broom, a shrubby little plant with bright red or yellow berries, is another great herbal tonic for congested veins and poor circulation.

Ginkgo biloba is a marvellous boost to memory and concentration because it stimulates the peripheral circulation to the brain. For the same reason, it can be a real ally in the battle to keep circulation steady and effective in the legs, and dozens of studies have shown its ability to do this, as well as to reduce discolouration. The Indian herb gotu kola works to strengthen blood vessel walls and improve blood flow through them. It is often combined with ginkgo, both herbs seemingly even more effective when used together than when working singly. Don't take ginkgo if you are on prescription drugs, as it can interact with them.

'Varicose veins are the result of an improper selection of grandparents.'
WILLIAM OSTLER, Canadian physician, 1849–1919

Defining idea...

Eat brightly coloured berries! They're rich in compounds that work to tone and strengthen the connective tissue that supports those vulnerable veins. Hawthorn is especially high in those healing compounds: take a 5ml teaspoon of a 1:5 tincture twice daily for three months, then give it a break for three weeks and repeat for another three months. If you've been working to improve your general circulatory health for those seven months, you should see a real difference. (Check with your doctor, though, if you are being treated for a heart condition.)

The jolly bright orange flowers of marigold, rich in healing carotenoids, come to the rescue of varicose veins too. Traditionally, marigold (usually known as calendula) ointment was rubbed gently into the legs of sufferers at night-time, using an upward movement, and bandaged into place. Over weeks of this treatment, inflammation and swelling subside, tissues are tautened, blood flow improves. Or you can make a strong tea using the dried marigold heads which can be ordered from a herbal supplier. Pour 500ml of boiling water over 4–5 flower heads, and leave to infuse for fifteen minutes, then strain. Use some of this night and morning to swab your legs (throw it away after two to three days, though).

How did it go?

Q I've read that you can use essential oils to help deal with varicose veins. Is this so?

A *Indeed it is; cypress, lavender, rosemary, geranium and juniper can all be helpful. To make a massage oil, add 10 drops of cypress, 10 of lavender or geranium and 5 of rosemary or juniper to 28g of a good carrier oil such as almond, and mix well. Stroke the oil gently into your legs using upward strokes – and no pressure – two or three times a day. Remember that essential oils should never be taken internally, though.*

Q My piles don't always bother me, but sometimes they're agony. Can you give me any suggestions for something that might help?

A *Sorting out constipation is a priority. Hard stools make matters worse; so does the pushing and straining that is a morning ritual for so many people, and which puts further pressure on the walls of the anus. Add much more fibre from fruit and vegetables to your diet - do that gradually – and retrain your toilet habits, and things will gradually improve. Meanwhile, two great remedies. The modest yellow-flowered lesser celandine was nicknamed pilewort by country people: the herb for piles. As you'd expect, pilewort ointment does a grand soothing job. So does marigold ointment; put a good dollop on three to four layers of tissue, apply it to your piles and leave it in place for a few hours.*

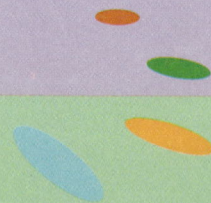

32

Piling on the pressure

As many as one in three of us in the Western world suffers from high blood pressure.

And most of the experts agree: it's a lifestyle disease.

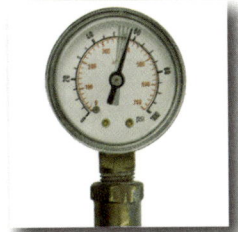

If you're living on junky fast food, taking no or minimal exercise, and letting stress really get to you, all the pills in the world won't be a lot of help. And don't expect herbs to fix it, either.

Since high blood pressure is potentially a killer, your doctor may want to put you on necessary medication immediately. But it's the lifestyle changes you make yourself – taking more exercise, practising relaxation, lowering caffeine and alcohol intake, losing some weight if you need to and adopting a seriously healthy diet – that will return you to health in the long run. Enlist some valuable herbs to help matters along. If you don't have high blood pressure, they'll help make sure you never develop it.

Hawthorn is an invigorating and nourishing tonic for the heart, improving function generally. It lowers blood pressure by relaxing and dilating artery walls, and although it's no quick fix for dangerously high blood pressure, it will work gently over months and years to improve matters. In Germany, where they are much more open to herbal medicine than anywhere else in the West, hundreds of doctors

Here's an idea for you...

Good news travels fast, and everybody now knows that dark chocolate is great for you. It's packed with healthy phenols, that's why, and the darker the chocolate, the higher the phenol content. But in the US study that produced this cheery finding, a quite significant drop in blood pressure was produced on a daily dose of just *one* of the sixteen squares in one of those big bars. More is not better. And don't expect a nice creamy comforting cup of drinking chocolate to do the trick: the milk will stop your body absorbing those phenols.

routinely prescribe it for their hypertensive patients. It's an outstandingly safe and non-toxic herb. If you're already on medication, though, discuss it with your doctor before starting to take it.

Limeflower tea calms anxiety and tension, helps relax muscles and arteries and is a friend to the heart and circulatory system generally. Yarrow is another excellent tonic for the circulation, and it can play a useful role in lowering blood pressure. Make up your own half-and-half mix of these dried herbs, and infuse a teaspoon in a mug of boiling water, covered, for five minutes, then strained. A daily cup could make a serious contribution to keeping your blood pressure normal.

Wonder-working garlic can help lower blood pressure. Like hawthorn, the effect is not dramatic, but why quibble? Garlic delivers such huge benefits for our general health that you'd think any sane person would be eating it regularly anyway. To help lower blood pressure, raw is better than cooked. Two cautions before you start mainlining on garlic. First, avoid it if you are on blood-thinning drugs like warfarin, since garlic, too, can thin your blood slightly: a healthy side effect for most of us. Secondly, it may irritate your stomach and give you heartburn, in which case you probably won't want to touch the stuff.

Some people thrive on life in the fast lane. But if it's your demanding, stressful multitasking life that's causing your rocketing blood pressure, two herbs can help you unwind and soothe your frazzled nerves. One of them is passionflower, which happens to be my own

'If you are not ready to change your way of living, you cannot be helped.'
HIPPOCRATES

Defining idea...

favourite remedy for sleeplessness, taken an hour or two before bedtime. The other is valerian, every doctor's favourite tranquilliser before Valium was invented. Both are often found in herbalists' blends for stress or sleeplessness. One thing you should know: valerian may not work for you, and those suffering from depression should not take it.

When herbalist Michael McIntyre sees patients with high blood pressure, he recommends lots of herbs and vegetables in their daily diet to maintain a healthy heart, blood pressure and circulatory system. 'Garlic, onions and scallions [spring onions] are excellent, and the rawer the better. Celery can help to lower blood pressure, and like dandelion leaves (delicious in salads) has a diuretic effect that helps to lower arterial pressure. Watercress is a circulatory stimulant. Use fresh or dried thyme, basil and rosemary in your cooking, and plenty of spices – cinnamon, cloves, turmeric, chilli and black pepper, ginger – all terrific for the cardiovascular system. Go for technicoloured food: dark green vegetables, tomatoes, red and yellow peppers, beetroot and all the bright berries – mulberries, elderberries, blueberries, hawthorn berries: the flavonoids that give colour to fruit and vegetables act as antioxidants, and confer tremendous benefit on the heart and blood vessels.'

How did it go?

Q   **I'm a coffee junkie, and my doctor tells me I simply must cut down on all that caffeine. I don't know what to drink instead. Are there any seriously drinkable herb teas?**

A   *Try hibiscus: it's a lovely dark red colour, and it has a full, pleasant taste, further improved by a spot of honey. In one small study, subjects drinking hibiscus tea for breakfast for some weeks had significant reductions in their blood pressure: controls taking a conventional vasodilator drug did only slightly better. The tea was made with 2 teaspoons of dried hibiscus covered with 500ml boiling water and allowed to steep for ten minutes. You can also buy teabags. Worth a try: it's non-toxic anyway.*

Q   **Somebody told me that olive leaf is good for people with high blood pressure. Is this actually true?**

A   *There's no hard evidence from clinical trials in human beings that this is so, although there has been some research in animals suggesting that it might be. But olive leaf has other benefits: it's high in antioxidants, among other things, so you might try taking it for a couple of weeks before you next have your blood pressure measured, to see if it improves matters at all. However, it can be irritating to the gut lining, so take it with a full meal.*

33

Hearty health

It's a lot easier to keep your heart healthy than to mend matters once the damage is done.

Get to know some herbs that will help maintain this mighty muscle in good shape.

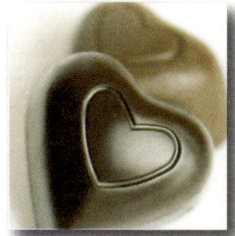

If you are already being treated for serious heart problems, you should discuss any herbal remedies you want to take as well with your doctor: there could be interactions or overlap.

But even if you are already on medication, there's plenty you can do to prevent further deterioration and even undo some of the damage. A professional herbalist will advise you on a herb regime tailored directly for you, and will be used to working alongside conventional doctors. Herbalists can call on a repertory of herbs that can protect you from heart disease, help sort out existing heart problems and prevent further damage if you are already at risk.

First and foremost, though, they'll impress on you the crucial importance of diet. America's Dr Dean Ornish has proved that heart damage can not only be prevented but actually reversed on a diet based on fresh fruit and vegetables, wholegrains, nuts and seeds, from which red meat, alcohol, white flour and white sugar are excluded. Fish oils – containing omega-3 fats essential to the heart – are a must. So are exercise and proper relaxation.

Here's an idea for you...

Take two spices – ginger and turmeric – and enjoy them in your cooking as often as you can. Both are rich in antioxidants, to combat the oxidative stress that may be putting your heart at risk. And both work to protect your arteries from the inflammation which researchers now believe may be the trigger for many a heart attack.

High on any herbalist's list of herbs for the heart is hawthorn. For the last two centuries, doctors the world over have been prescribing this beautiful hedgerow herb for heart problems, and no wonder. It works to strengthen and steady the heartbeat, increase blood flow to the heart by dilating the coronary arteries and it helps protect you from a heart attack. It's an outstandingly safe herb which can be taken for years on end, with only very rare and mild side effects. According to herbalist Dr Ann Walker, 'it is possible that taken for a long period of time, hawthorn may even regress established atheromas – those fatty plaques in your arteries which spell trouble. And if you don't have a heart condition, and you're getting on and feel you should be doing something for your heart, hawthorn is an excellent preventative.'

Ginkgo biloba has made a name for itself as a protector of the ageing brain. By the same token, it's good news for heart health too. Very rich in antioxidants to protect against oxidative damage to the heart, it helps keeps veins relaxed and open and protects against stroke. It's an excellent supplement for the elderly, for both reasons, though you shouldn't take it if you're already on medication for blood or other disorders. If I already had a heart problem, I'd want to discuss it with my herbalist, too.

Garlic's benefits for the heart and circulation have been studied in literally thousands of research projects. Just what can it do? Well, its chief role is to help keep your aorta – the body's chief artery – young and supple, to avoid the dangerous stiffening that often comes with age. It helps prevent the blood clotting that can be a forerunner of dangerous strokes and, once clots have formed, it can help break them down in the blood. It can also help gently lower blood pressure, though it may take time to do this. The best way to take garlic is to eat it raw – what foodie would want to replace this fantastic stuff with a mere capsule? But if you really can't bear the taste, take it in pill form. Because of its blood-thinning tendency, people taking anticoagulants or anti-platelet drugs should avoid garlic: your doctor will advise you on this. And prolonged heavy dosing should be avoided in pregnancy – though breastfed babies seem to love the taste.

'Go as far back in time as you like, and you'll find that through the length and breadth of Europe, hawthorn has always been considered the greatest of the "protective plants".'
JEAN PALAISEUL, *Grandmother's Secrets*

Defining idea...

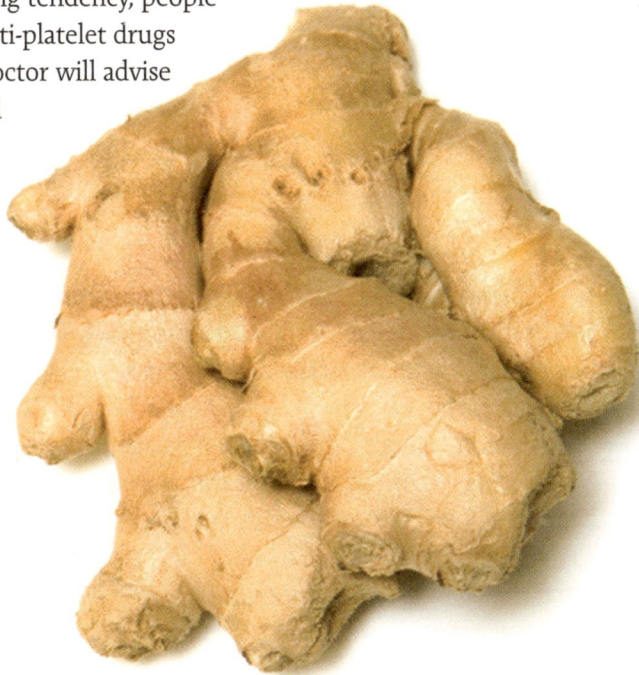

141

How did it go?

Q **I suffer from palpitations, and my doctor gives me tablets for my heart condition which help. Is there something herbal I can do as well?**

A *Make sure your diet provides plenty of calcium and magnesium, especially the latter. One herb specific for this condition, points out Ann Walker, is motherwort, a superb sedative for the nerves and heart. 'Drink motherwort tea', runs an old saying, 'and live to be a source of continuous astonishment and frustration to your heirs.' Motherwort is often combined with limeflowers and lemon balm in equal parts. Stock up on all three and brew yourself a cupful of hearty health two or three times a day. To make it put 2 teaspoons in a cupful of boiling water and infuse, covered, for fifteen minutes.*

Q **I'm on medication for my heart, but I feel that one of the problems is that I get stressed, upset and angry very easily. Is there something you can suggest to help me calm down and unwind?**

A *Doctors in Ancient Greece and Rome recommended valerian for any kind of nervous trouble, and over centuries it has built a reputation as a first-class calmer of nervous disorders such as stress, anxiety, sleeplessness and tension. It works on the central nervous system, and researchers have rated it as effective as the chemical tranquillisers developed last century, though it has few or none of their dodgy side effects. It can also be used in daytime since it doesn't cause drowsiness. But it doesn't work for everyone, and it's not for those suffering from depression. A good alternative is passionflower.*

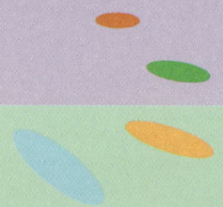

34

Flu-struck

When there's flu around, beef up your immune defences with some effective herbs.

And if you fall a victim, trust them to see you through.

Flu symptoms can include fever, a general achiness, headache, cough, sore throat and a bone-deep tiredness. You'll start to feel rotten up to four days after the virus has hit you – but like the common cold, it needs to be dealt with at the very first ache or shiver if you're going to get on top of it. Stay in bed, rest, drink plenty of hot lemon with ginger and honey.

At my convent boarding school, all those years ago, we were dosed with cinnamon and quinine if we looked like coming down with something nasty. This was standard treatment: up to the 1950s or 60s, any high-street chemist would have suggested cinnamon in large doses for a case of flu, because of its antiseptic and warming properties. Cinnamon is actually one of the great antiseptics, I learned years later. In the great flu pandemics of the early twentieth century, which killed millions of people, a Dr Joseph Ross of Manchester claimed to have saved the lives of hundreds of patients with his Cinnamon Treatment. If they began taking it within the first day, they were usually over the flu within two days, five at the outside.

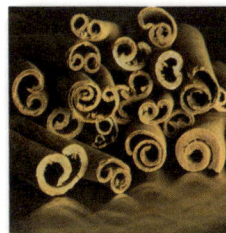

Here's an idea for you...

Hot cayenne pepper delivers a terrific boost to the immune system and warms you right through. Invest in a little bottle of *capsicum* tincture, and when you're feeling low, chilly and vulnerable, add a quarter of a teaspoon to a drink of hot lemon and honey. (Make sure the bottle is well-labelled, though, and keep out of reach of children!)

To try Dr Ross's treatment, you will need 75g of good quality cinnamon bark and a 75cl bottle of any old brandy. Pack the cinnamon quills into the bottle and leave them to macerate for a week to ten days. At the very first ache or shiver of a cold or flu, take 1–2 teaspoonfuls in 2 tablespoons of hot water half-hourly for two hours, then hourly until your temperature is normal. If you want to avoid alcohol, heat equal quantities of the brandy and water in a pan for a few minutes: the alcohol will evaporate off. You can also use this as prevention: when there's flu around, take a daily dose in hot water at bedtime.

Like the cinnamon treatment, echinacea needs to be taken at the very first sign of flu, with regularly repeated doses. Don't economise here – buy your echinacea from a reputable herbal supplier. A good product, of sufficient strength, will make your tongue tingle a little: it's the echinacea trademark, and nothing to worry about. Better still, use echinacea at a lower dose as prevention: take it regularly through the flu season.

Keep some tincture of boneset on hand when the flu season looms; it's one of the first herbs a herbalist would turn to. This was a remedy learned by settlers in North America from the natives, and it earned its name because it helps relieve the bone-deep aching of classic flu. Take it at the first signs; it's a wonderful remedy for the assorted aches, pains and general misery, and it's a mild stimulant to the immune system, as well. Boneset promotes gentle perspiration to help you throw off the infection and it needs to be drunk hot, so add the suggested dose of tincture to a nice comforting hot drink – perhaps freshly squeezed lemon in a mugful of boiling water with a little honey. Drink it in bed three times a day.

'There is a remedy for every illness to be found in nature.'
HIPPOCRATES

Defining idea…

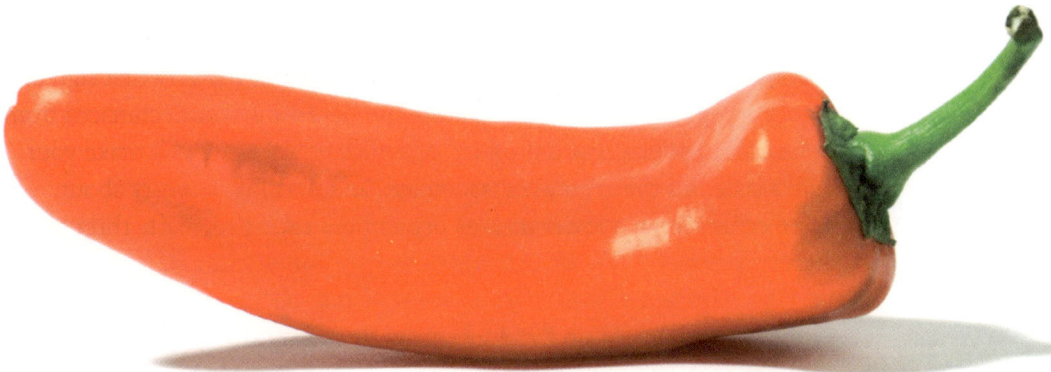

145

How did it go?

Q My husband swears by a hot bedtime grog to rout a virus – whisky, orange juice and an aspirin. Any comments?

A   *Not a bad idea at all, but you can make a much more potent one. Dr Jean Valnet, the French founding father of modern aromatherapy, suggested the following to his patients: A tot of whisky, to which is added half a squeezed lemon, a tablespoonful of honey, and a large glass of hot water in which a small piece of cinnamon and a clove have been boiled for two to three minutes. Leave to infuse for twenty minutes. Both cinnamon and cloves are warming, stimulating and antiseptic.*

Q Is there anything that can really help get you through the flu fast?

A   *Elderberries have a long folk reputation as a cold and flu remedy, so Dr Madeleine Mumcuoglu, an Israeli virologist, decided to test an extract of elderberry against the actual virus. She discovered that the influenza virus invades cells by puncturing their walls with the tiny spikes of hemaglutinin that cover its surface: the active ingredient in elderberry disables the spikes by binding to them. A study published by the* Journal of Alternative and Complementary Medicine *found that nearly 90% of flu patients given the elderberry preparation were completely free of symptoms within two to three days, compared to at least six days with a placebo. It's important to note that the elderberry patients were taking 15ml doses four times a day: just a glug or a single pill of even the most potent remedy isn't going to see off a persistent virus. Dr. Mumcuoglu's elderberry extract is now widely on sale.*

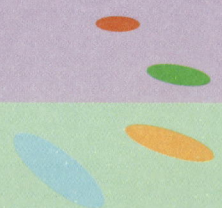

35

Viral load

Noticed how there's always 'a virus going round' these days?

If you don't want to be one of the victims, look to your defences now.

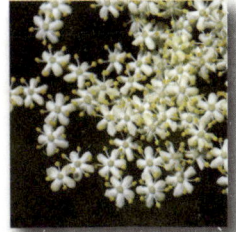

Good immune defences depend on a healthy outlook as well as healthy living. Add in a good nourishing diet, enough sleep, regular exercise, and your resistance should be top level. If you're still falling prey to any passing bug, call on some powerful herbal help.

The foremost herbal immune booster is popular echinacea. Dozens of clinical studies have established that echinacea acts to enhance immune activity in a number of ways, and if you are chesty and an easy victim to winter colds, coughs and bronchitis, take echinacea daily through the winter months; double the dose at the first sign of trouble.

'Elderflowers are our own echinacea,' says Scottish herbalist Dee Atkinson of Napier's. She puts them both into an echinacea and elderflower compound, together with sage and other antiseptic herbs, which clients take for added protection when there are bugs around.

Here's an idea for you...

In his book *Herbal Antibiotics*, US herbalist Stephen Harrod Buhner suggests the 'Best Cold and Flu Tea'. Use 2 teaspoons of sage, the juice of a lemon (or a teaspoon of lemon balm), a pinch of cayenne pepper and a tablespoon of honey. Pour a cup of boiling water over the sage (and the lemon balm, if you're using that) and allow it to steep for ten minutes. Then strain out the herbs, add the remaining ingredients and drink the tea hot.

The elder tree in fact supplies a whole range of popular country medicines, particularly as a cold and flu preventive. Elderflowers gently stimulate the immune response, and they have antiviral activity. Keep a packet of elderflower tea bags in your store cupboard for a protective hot – and delicious – bedtime drink when there are colds around, or have a bottle of ready-made elderflower cordial to hand. Elderberry wines and cordials used to be made all over Europe in autumn when the little black berries appeared. They were drunk hot to help ward off colds or flu bugs.

Another great friend to the immune system is Siberian ginseng. Numbers of studies, carried out over several decades with thousands of subjects, have shown how it can boost resistance to disease, as well as to stress in any form and aid convalescence. In one study, 1000 factory workers were given a daily dose of Siberian ginseng for two winter months; they had almost two-and-a-half times fewer flu or acute respiratory infections than a matched group of controls. Siberian ginseng can safely be taken for as long as six weeks, but then you should take a fortnight's break before starting up again. Don't take it, by the way, if you have an acute infection or if you are on digoxin for your heart.

Garlic has legendary antiseptic powers, working against bacteria, viruses and fungi alike: its antiseptic action is greatest when it is eaten raw, so crunch a finely chopped clove of it whenever you make a salad. Some friends of mine chop up three or four cloves of garlic and eat them in a sandwich with thickly buttered bread when they feel a cold coming on. It works, they say, so you may want to give it a try. Onions, close relatives of garlic, have considerable antiviral powers of their own, so include plenty of onions in your winter diet too: chopped up raw in salads, or added to soups and casseroles. And don't forget that thyme, rosemary, sage and oregano are all powerfully antiseptic: use them regularly when you're cooking.

'Serious illness doesn't bother me for long because I am too inhospitable a host.'
ALBERT SCHWEITZER

Defining idea...

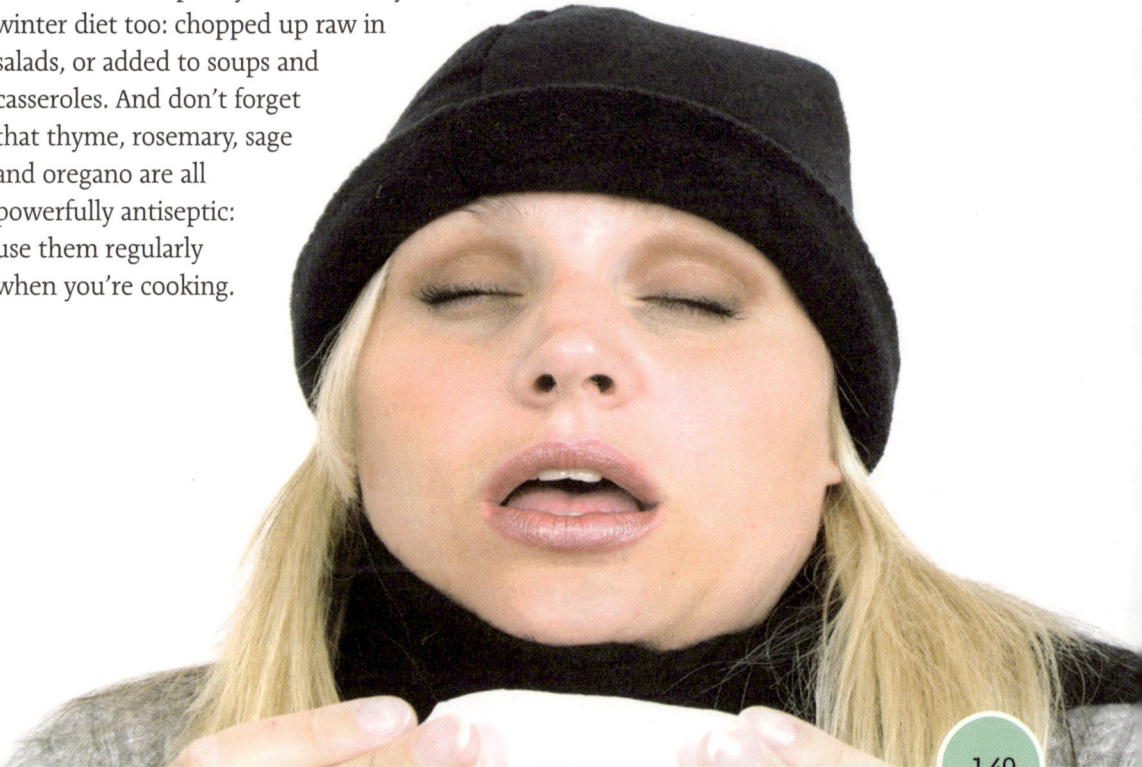

149

How did
it go?

Q   I thought magic mushrooms just gave you a nice high, but I've heard about three magic mushrooms for health. Is this right?

A   *The mushrooms you heard about may not be magic, but they're pretty marvellous: they're from Asia, and they are called reishi, maitake and shiitake. They won't give you a high but these three are used in medicine in China and Japan, and they are considered powerful tonics for the immune system. Researchers in these countries and in the US have identified compounds in these magic mushrooms that beef up the immune system in a number of important ways. One of the three – shiitake – can be found at plenty of greengrocers and supermarkets. Enjoy these dark brown mushrooms with the distinctive up-front taste in soups, stews, salads, omelettes or pasta sauces.*

Q   Are there any other wonderful immune-boosters in Chinese medicine?

A   *Certainly; improving general health and resistance is a priority. The most highly valued plants – and those, incidentally, which are safest to take long term – are the great tonic herbs which act not so much to counteract specific disease states as to correct deficiencies and enhance general vitality and resistance. In this age of superbugs and terrifying new plagues, what could make more sense? The supreme Chinese tonic herb is ginseng, but good ginseng is very expensive. Another is astragalus root, which has been intensively studied by Western scientists. They found that it has an impressive range of immune-activating properties. 'The conclusion being drawn by most Western herbalists,' comments leading US herbal authority David Hoffmann, 'is that astragalus is an ideal remedy for anyone who might be immuno-compromised in any way. This can range from someone who easily catches cold to someone with cancer.' Astragalus is extremely safe, with no known toxicity or adverse effects.*

36

Horrible herpes

As anyone who has ever suffered it knows, there's not much doctors can do to ease the pain of shingles.

But don't despair: herbs offer plenty of hope to its victims.

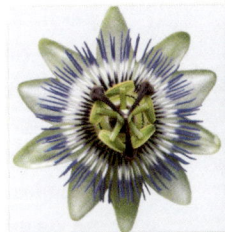

Remember getting chickenpox all those years ago? The varicella zoster virus which caused it has been lying dormant in your nerve endings ever since. At times of great stress, or when the immune system is at a specially low ebb – during cancer chemotherapy, for instance – the virus can spring to life and start replicating, travelling along the nerves until it reaches the skin's surface first as a painful red rash, then as a crop of tiny blisters. This is shingles – *herpes zoster* – and you wouldn't wish it on your worst enemy, especially when it lingers on for months, even years sometimes, after the last scab has dropped off.

Your doctor may prescribe one of a small handful of antiviral drugs, with creams to apply to the painful lesions. But when it comes to relieving the pain, the stress and the depression caused by this unpleasant condition, herbal medicine can make a huge difference. Don't forget, always tell your doctor if you are taking herbal medicines at the same time as prescription drugs, in case there might be an interaction.

Here's an idea for you...

If the pain and misery are wrecking your sleep, try passionflower, effective for just those times when agitated nerves keep you tossing and turning. It helps relieve nerve-related pain such as that of shingles, too. Passionflower – on its own or combined with other sedative herbs such as hops or valerian – is a common ingredient in herbal sleep remedies.

Your immune system is hugely in need of support, and a good echinacea should be taken throughout the illness.

Shingles directly attacks nerves, and the pain can be excruciating. St John's wort (*Hypericum perforatum*) is almost specific for nerve pain, while its well-known antidepressant effect will help lift the spirits of the sufferer, and its antiviral action may help see off the *herpes zoster* virus responsible. Herbalists have successfully treated shingles patients with St John's wort combined with echinacea to bolster the sagging immune system. The preparation of St John's wort they use is one standardised to a high level of the most active ingredient, hypericin. (Don't take St John's wort if you are on prescription medication.)

When applied topically, St John's wort has an analgesic effect, as well as healing and anti-inflammatory qualities which make it especially helpful. Herbalist Jill Davies suggests mixing the beautiful red oil of St John's wort with equal parts of aloe vera gel and witch hazel gel, and applying it up to five times daily, letting it dry before replacing clothing. Both witch hazel and aloe vera gels cool and soothe. Calendula, the great healer, works well here too: combine equal parts of St John's wort and calendula tinctures, dilute with the same amount of water, and swab the agonising lesions.

Australian herbalist Robyn Kirby suggests combining 25ml each of the tinctures of St John's wort and plantain, another great healing plant. Combine this mix with equal parts of water, she suggests in her book *Herbs for Healing*, and dab on the rash with cotton wool until the pain is eased. St John's wort ointment or the oil can also be used on areas which are no longer red and blistered but still painful.

'Pain addeth zest unto pleasure, and teacheth the luxury of health.'
MARTIN FARQUHAR TUPPER, writer and poet

Defining idea...

Dr Jean Valnet, the founding father of modern aromatherapy, developed a special mix of pure, organically produced essential oils which he christened Tegarome. It contained lavender, thyme, sage, eucalyptus, rosemary and cypress – calming, analgesic and antiviral in their actions. Apply the neat oil on compresses over affected areas, to be bandaged or taped loosely into place, and apply fresh compresses every three to four hours if possible. Patients also take magnesium supplements and pain is usually greatly diminished within a day or two. Dr Valnet said of the Tegarome treatment: 'We have not yet recorded a single failure in twenty-five years among countless cases treated within the first fifteen to twenty days in this way.' Remember that essential oils should not be taken internally and keep them away from your eyes.

American-based herbalist David Hoffmann points out that in shingles 'the nervous system needs as much help as it can get' – nervine tonics to 'feed' the traumatised nerve tissue and nervine relaxants to lessen associated anxiety or tension. He suggests oats as a tonic for the nerves, and St John's wort as both tonic and relaxant, as well as supplements of vitamin B complex and vitamin C. The two are often combined in over-the-counter herbal products.

153

How did it go?

Q   Someone told me they'd heard that ordinary tea can help shingles. Is this really so?

A   *They heard right. A Harley Street doctor found that much the most successful topical treatment for painful shingles was Earl Grey tea. Patents are now being sought for a variety of ingenious applications: creams, sprays, lotions, etc. Meanwhile, just brew up a cup of Earl Grey tea, let it cool and swab it on – or apply the cooled tea bag. Aromatherapists aren't surprised by this: they use bergamot oil for a range of skin problems, including chickenpox and cold sores (both herpes problems), and it's that trace of bergamot oil which gives Earl Grey tea its special taste.*

Q   The local chemist suggested a cream made from chilli peppers. Sounds unbelievable – could this really help?

A   *It might sound like putting out fire with fire, but yes, apparently it can. Researchers found that the cream brings genuine relief both in the acute phase of shingles and for the pain - sometimes even worse - which can persist long after the worst is over. It works, apparently, by blocking pain signals from nerve endings to the brain, so that you no longer experience the pain. Chemists can supply capsaicin cream at two concentrations: 0.025% for acute pain and slightly stronger - 0.05% - for lingering pain. Try the lowest but be warned - it may take some getting used to! And don't forget to wash your hands after applying it, either.*

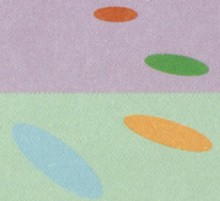

37

Getting over it

Convalescence? Now there's an old-fashioned word for you.

Nobody does convalescence any more: we're all much too busy getting back to our rushed, demanding lifestyles again.

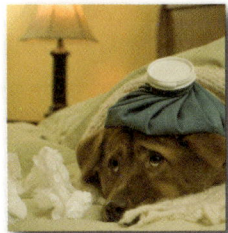

Even if you're able to take time off to recover in bed, there may be nobody around to minister to you. But a bout of flu, an attack of bronchitis, even a heavy cold can all leave your immune defences in rags. Give yourself a break. Your body needs time and tender loving care to get itself up and running again. Toning, nourishing and stimulating herbs can be real friends at such times. And some of the most helpful will already be at hand, in your own kitchen.

Cinnamon has awesome antiseptic powers but it's also a wonderful tonic, especially for people worn out by battling a bug. Trust the French to come up with this delicious way of exploiting its powers: in a wine, to be drunk hot and comforting. To make it, take a litre of a good, sweetish white wine, add 10 mint leaves and 25g cinnamon bark, broken into shavings. Stopper the bottle and leave to infuse for three days, then strain and drink an occasional small glassful, heated. If you want to stay off the alcohol, let it simmer gently for ten to fifteen minutes and the alcohol will evaporate.

Here's an idea for you...

Barley water was another Victorian sick-room staple and with reason: this marvellous grain helps restore energy, revive appetite, rebuild strength and generally speed recovery from that debilitating illness. It helps heal inflammatory conditions right through the gut. And it's also rich in vitamins and minerals, especially iron and B vitamins. To make it, put 50g of unrefined pot barley in a pan with 600ml of water, bring to the boil and simmer for thirty minutes. Add 1 1/2 tablespoons of honey and stir well. Cool, strain, add the juice of half a lemon and drink it, lukewarm, throughout the day.

The famous German herbalist Abbe Kneipp described oats as 'an excellent restorative for convalescents exhausted by serious illness', and no modern herbalist would disagree. When you're feeling too knackered to cook a proper meal, go for a bowl of porridge, with a little cream and honey. It's made in minutes, is highly nourishing, easily digested, high in B vitamins, rich in useful minerals like iron and zinc, and a wonderful pick-me-up to the whole nervous system. Herbalists use a juice or tincture made from the whole green plant when it is just flowering for an even better nerve tonic: look for *Avena sativa* in blends at a herbal supplier.

Stress and exhaustion are nothing new; nineteenth-century Edinburgh herbalist Duncan Napier saw plenty of patients suffering from just that. He made up for them what he called his Nerve Debility Tonic, in which oats were a key ingredient. You can still buy it today from the herbal shops named after him. Now renamed Skullcap, Oat and Passionflower, it's an all-round tonic for nerves, digestion and the immune system – all likely to be in need of a little something to buck them up after a bout of flu. Another ingredient is gentian, from the roots of that pretty blue Alpine flower, a bitter herb that not only improves digestion and appetite, but can do wonders for the post-flu blues.

Slippery elm was a great Victorian favourite for convalescence – one of the most useful remedies taught to European settlers by North American Indians. It's actually the inner bark of the American elm, and it's dried and powdered for use. To prepare it, take a teaspoon of the powder, make it into a paste with cold water, and pour on a cupful of boiling water, stirring all the time. Easily assimilated, it's especially useful if your digestive system is affected, as so often in illness, because the soft mucilage it contains is very healing for an irritated gut. You may find it a bit bland: add a little honey and powdered cinnamon.

'Sickness comes on horseback, but departs on foot.'
Dutch proverb.

Defining idea…

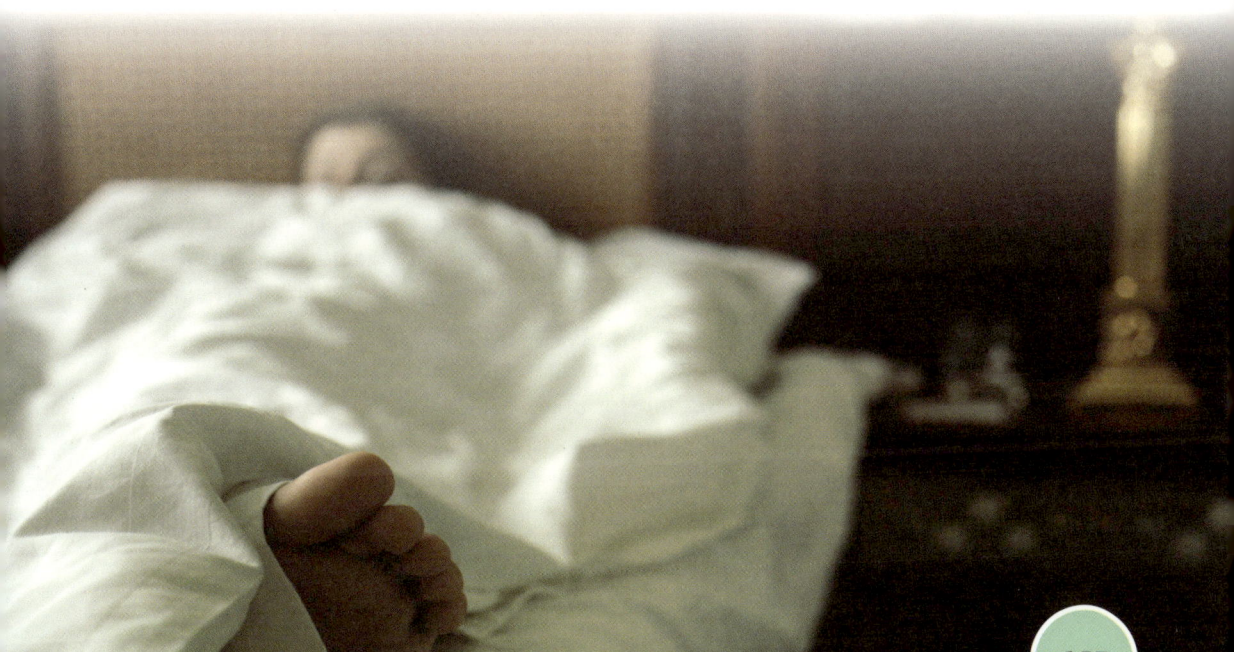

How did it go?

Q I've been in bed for ten days with nasty bronchitis, and although I know I need the sleep badly, I simply find myself lying awake for hours. Can you suggest something I might use?

A *Try passionflower: it's a gentle but extremely effective sleep-inducer, exerting a sedative effect on strung-up nerves. Take a dose of the tincture about an hour before you plan going to bed, and you should sleep sweetly and soundly, with no chemical hangover the next morning. In made-up remedies it is often combined with sedative hops, or with the rather more powerful valerian.*

Q I'm getting over a nasty viral infection, and though I've had to go back to work, I live on my own and simply don't have the energy to shop for nourishing food, let alone spend time cooking it. I'm just living on cartons of soup and bread and cheese. I feel I ought to be eating better than this – but how?

A *Fifteen years ago, US herbalist Richard Schulze had many patients severely ill, or slowly getting over serious disease, and in the same boat as you. He devised a powdered green superfood for them, now known as Dr Richard Schulze's Superfood Plus. It's highly nutritious, needing only two minutes' preparation, and needing almost no digestion. Among its ingredients are mineral-rich algae spirulina and chlorella, the seaweed dulse, barley and wheat grass, any one of which would be a huge nutritional plus. It can be ordered online.*

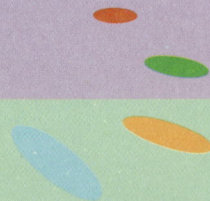

38

Down in the mouth

Horrid little mouth ulcers that make eating painful? Blisters on your tongue? Gum infections that give you sleepless nights?

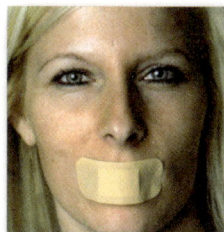

No wonder you feel down in the mouth. Cheer up: there are plenty of herbal answers.

Mouth ulcers spell regular trouble for millions of people. They appear without warning, make eating or drinking a misery and can hang around for days. Nobody knows exactly what causes them, but it's often possible to work out what the trigger is in your particular case. Chronic indigestion, perhaps? Heartburn? An overdose of a food to which you are sensitive, perhaps – too much wheat or dairy? A friend of mine ate oranges regularly for years as a source of the vitamin C she hoped might help clear her painful mouth ulcers – until a chance remark heard on the radio suggested that oranges might be the problem, not the solution. She stopped eating citrus fruit and has never had a mouth ulcer since.

Fluoride in toothpaste has been known to give some people mouth ulcers. So has the detergent used in just about every toothpaste – sodium laurel or laureth sulphate. Avoid these: shop for a 'green' toothpaste.

Here's an idea for you...

Cold sores (those unsightly little blisters on or around the lips) and painful genital herpes are both viral infections. A German study looked at a cream containing 1% lemon balm extract applied five times a day and used by people suffering from both these conditions. The results were interesting; 60% reported that their lesions had healed within four days; by the eighth day 96% were lesion-free. To make your own, add a teaspoonful of lemon balm tincture, or a few drops of the essential oil, to some aqueous cream from the chemist – and apply it.

A number of herbs are almost miraculously effective at soothing the pain, clearing up any infection and healing sore spots. Two in particular head my own list of tried-and-tested favourites: propolis and marigold.

Propolis is amazing stuff. It's composed of resins from various aromatic trees harvested by hardworking bees and plastered all around their hives to safeguard them from the infections that might otherwise sweep through their warm crowded homes. Dozens of studies have shown propolis to be extraordinarily effective against infections of the mouth and throat. This dark sticky stuff is supplied as a tincture, in dropper bottles, at good health food stores. Keep it handy if you're prone to mouth ulcers; at the very first sign, coat a cotton-wool bud in the tincture and apply it directly to the spot. It may sting a little at first, but it will provide fast relief, and clear the sore in short order. Reapply it several times a day, as necessary.

You can use a tincture of marigold – usually known as calendula – in the same way. Dilute a $^1/_2$ tsp of the tincture in a tablespoonful of warm water, and apply it directly to the sores.

The twinge that you assume is an aching tooth may well be the initial infection and inflammation of the gum surrounding it: treat this, and there may be no toothache to deal with. Toothache usually strikes late on a Friday evening, just as dentists are shutting up shop for the weekend. I was able to call my own homeopathic dentist during working hours, fortunately, when I was stricken in foreign parts. 'Buy some tincture of calendula,' he advised me. 'Soak swabs of cotton wool in the tincture, and pack them round the problem tooth all day and until you go to sleep at night. Your gum may feel a little numb, but the pain will go and hopefully the infection will clear.' By the next morning I didn't have toothache any more, and my family has been using this amazing first aid for toothache ever since.

'Faced with the choice of enduring a bad toothache or going to the dentist, we generally tried to ride out the bad tooth.'
JOSEPH BARBERA, US cartoon genius

Defining idea...

How did it go?

Q   I'm told that oil of cloves is an effective emergency treatment for toothache: do most chemists sell this, and how do you use it?

A   *Yes they do, and clove oil is especially helpful for toothache, since cloves work both as anaesthetic and as antiseptic. Put a little oil of cloves on your finger and apply it directly to the aching tooth or gum. If you don't have any oil of cloves, pick a clove or two from the jar in your spice rack and chew it gently, as near as you can bear to the throbbing tooth. Keep the clove in your mouth and replace it when it doesn't seem to be working any longer, but two cloves is enough of this potent medicine and should do the trick.*

Q   I read somewhere that myrrh is supposed to be good for mouth ulcers, and I'd like to try it if so. What is it, and how do I use it?

A   *Myrrh is prepared from the sticky resin that exudes from the myrrh bush and, like propolis, it is usually supplied by the chemist or health-food store as a tincture. It helps clear up infections and relieve inflammation. Apply the tincture neat to your mouth sores using a cotton-wool bud. It also makes a useful mouthwash which will make your breath more fragrant: add a teaspoonful of the tincture to a little warm water, and swish around your mouth for a minute or two. Regular use will help firm up your gums if they are in poor shape and protect your teeth from decay, so it's a frequent ingredient in good herbal mouthwashes.*

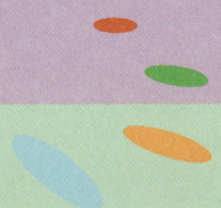

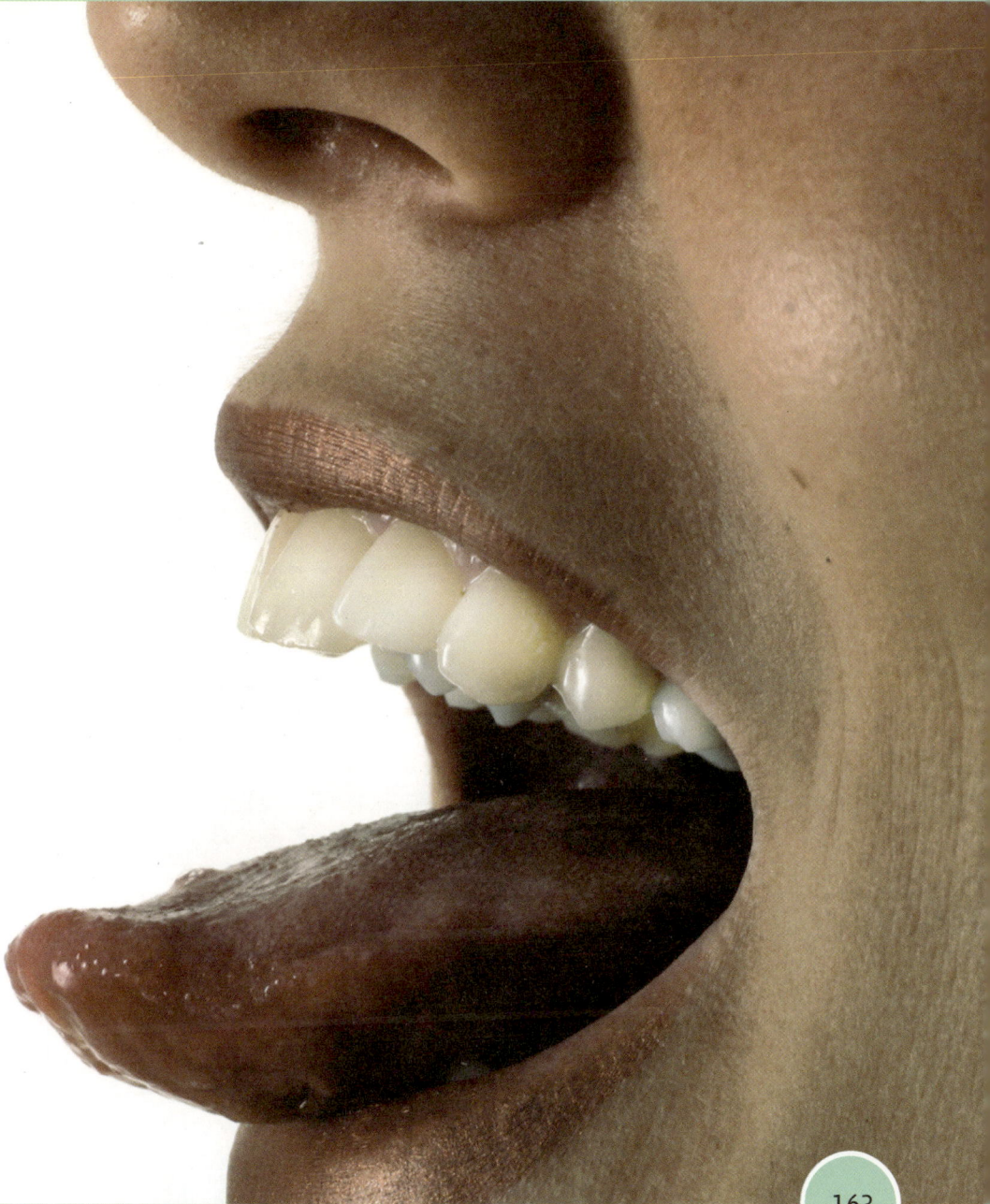

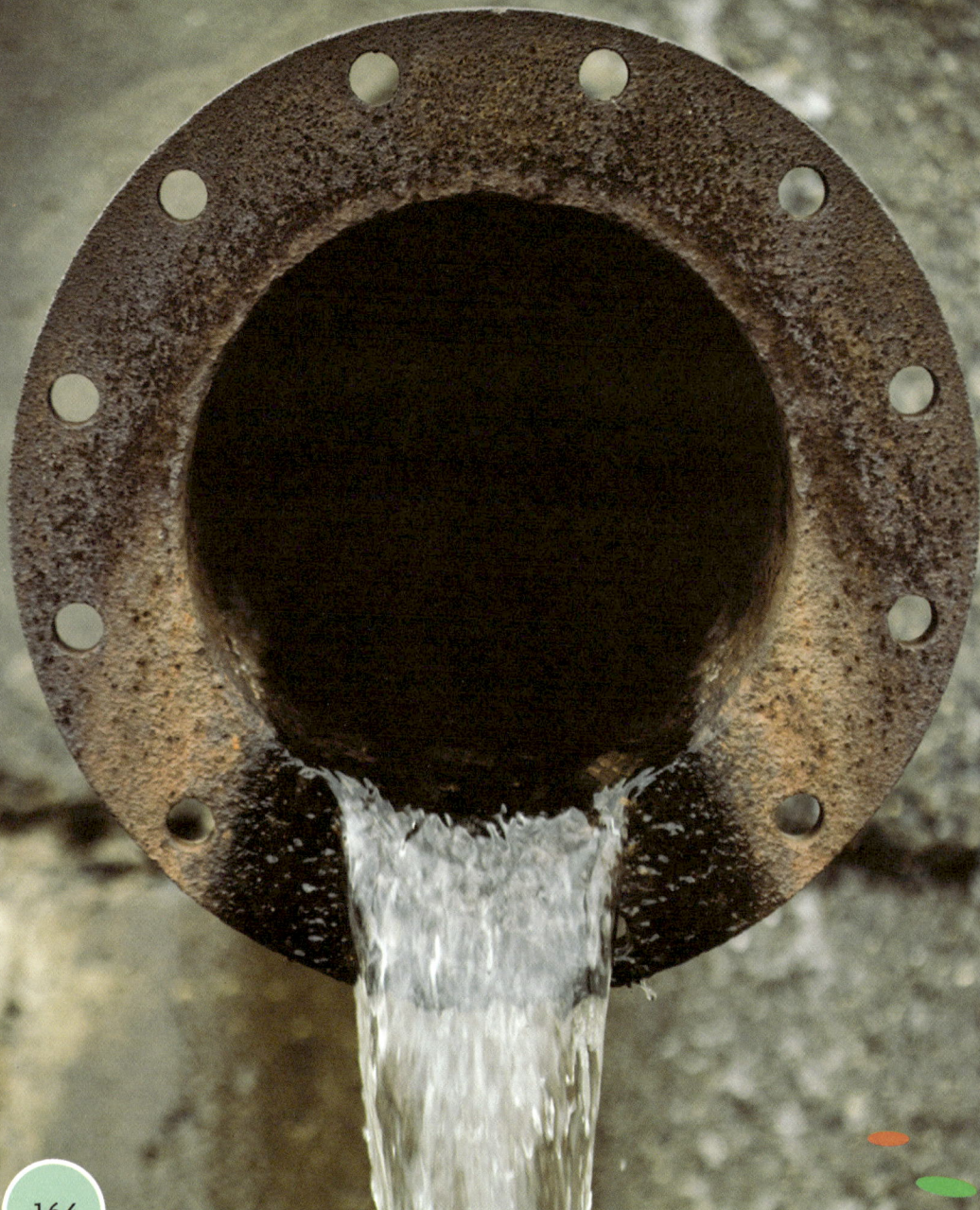

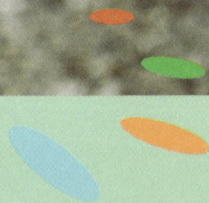

39

Waterworks

If you keep getting bouts of cystitis, the bugs that are responsible are probably becoming resistant to antibiotics.

Use herbs to clear up the infection, soothe the inflammation and help guard against further attacks.

Go to the doctor if you're running a fever, experiencing serious pain in your bladder or lower back, or noticing blood in your urine. They could indicate serious kidney problems.

Meanwhile, here are tried and trusted herbal remedies for urinary tract infections (UTI) – and one new star. That's cranberry, of course, the shiny red berries most of us only see as a sauce for festive roast turkey. But cranberry was a North American folk remedy for bladder infections long before scientific researchers took a close look at it. Now we know that cranberries contain a compound called arbutin. Once it enters the urine, arbutin splits into other compounds, one of which, hydroquinone, has a direct antiseptic action on the kidneys, the urinary tract and the bladder. Hydroquinone also plays a neat little trick on those E.coli bugs: it stops them anchoring to the wall of the urinary tract and, instead, they are washed away with the urine. In clinical trials, even drinking a commercial, highly sweetened cranberry juice helped clear infections. You can also buy unsweetened – very tart and rather pricey – cranberry juice, or tablets containing concentrated cranberry

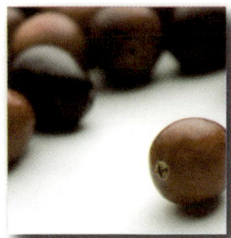

Here's an idea for you...

Why keep cranberries for Christmas? They're a superfood in their own right: no other fruit is higher in wonder-working antioxidants than the cranberry. While they're in season, stew them with apples, add them to frozen *frutti di bosco* mixes for great winter puddings or throw a small handful in the juicer along with half a dozen carrots and chunks of peeled raw beetroot for a wonderful tart pink pick-me-up. You'll be protecting yourself from urinary tract infections at the same time. And while they're in season and cheap at your greengrocer, why not toss two or three packs into your freezer?

extract. You can also add dried cranberries to a dried fruit compote. There have been some reports in the press about cranberry causing problems, but there's lots of really good research backing up its benefits for UTIs, so give it a try.

Bearberry, a close plant relation of cranberries, is one of the first remedies a herbalist would think of in treating this problem, and an ingredient in almost every herbal remedy for cystitis on the market. Guess what? It's arbutin at work again, plus other plant chemicals that will work to soothe, tone and strengthen your urinary tract, as well as seeing off those *E.coli* bugs.

Buchu is yet another herbal standby; its leaves contain bacteria-killing oils which will help clean up your urinary tract. It's especially useful when urinating causes a painful burning sensation, and marshmallow can be helpful here too, soothing and calming inflammation. Make up a herbal mix of buchu and marshmallow leaves and use it for a tea to be drunk three times a day while the infection persists. To make the tea, put a good teaspoon of the herbs in a mug, fill it with boiling water and infuse, covered, for ten minutes. Then strain and drink hot.

Infection weakens your urinary tract, which makes it much more vulnerable to further assaults. If this is the case, take a couple of doses of buchu from time to time as prevention, and give yourself a long course of a good herbal tonic. My favourite is a Swiss-made mix of healing herbs called Bio-Strath. Lemon balm, chamomile, elder, lavender, sage and thyme are among the herbs in this useful mix. In a number of clinical trials, it has proved its ability to boost resistance, raise energy levels and lift the spirits. It's prepared as a pleasant-tasting liquid: a couple of good glugs a day over four to six weeks will raise your resistance and improve your general health.

Defining idea...

'*Bladder infections are common in women: 10–20% of all women have urinary tract discomfort at least once a year, 37.5% of all women with no history of UTI will have one within ten years; 2.4% of healthy women have elevated bacteria in urine – unrecognised UTI.'*
JOSEPH PIZZORNO, MICHAEL MURRAY and HERB JOINER-BEY, in *The Clinician's Handbook of Natural Medicine*

How did it go?

Q **Is there anything else I should be drinking to help my cystitis?**

A *Yes: plenty of water! If you aren't drinking enough water to keep those kidneys busy flushing through your urinary tract, these remedies can't do their stuff. So drink, drink and then drink some more, at least a litre a day if possible. (Refill a litre-sized mineral water bottle every morning, and aim to empty it before you go to bed.) Sorry, but tea and coffee don't count as part of your water intake here; nor do fizzy drinks, while alcohol actually irritates your poor kidneys. Drink plenty of chamomile tea, on the other hand: it's recommended for cystitis. You can also use the cold tea as a cooling, soothing wash for the whole area. Barley water, home-made from unrefined pot barley, is good, too.*

Q **I hate the taste of cranberries. Are there any other fruits that might work for cystitis?**

A *Yes, indeed. Try bilberries, a European folk remedy for cystitis long before cranberries ever crossed the Atlantic. It turns out they also contain arbutin, the wonder-working compound in cranberries, and the two berries actually belong to the same plant family – you will probably find blueberries, the bilberry's cultivated relative, more easily. France's Dr Jean Valnet suggested to his patients that they put a handful of bilberries in a litre of water, bring to the boil and simmer for five minutes, then let it steep for another ten minutes. The liquid was strained, pressing out as much of the remaining juice in the berries as possible, then drunk three times a day.*

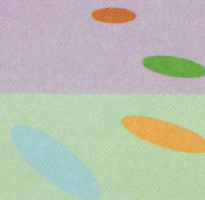

40

Out of joint

Arthritis may be the oldest disease on the planet: typical signs of wear and tear show up even on dinosaur skeletons.

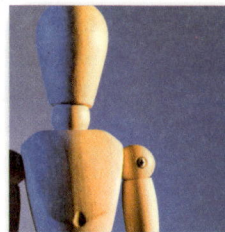

So human beings have had plenty of time to work out which plants might help soothe their aching joints. Here are some of the best.

Roman armies, on frontier duty in Britain 2000 years ago, suffered miseries from the cold damp climate, so unlike warm, sunny Italy. Solution: their army surgeons brought the seeds of wild nettles to Britain to plant around their camps. Then they prescribed the stinging treatment: flogging swollen joints with the nettles. Believe it or not, many arthritic patients today still practise nettle-sting therapy.

In a small study carried out at the UK's Southampton University, stinging nettle leaves were applied to the hands of twenty-seven osteoarthritis sufferers daily for a week. At the end of the trial, fourteen of them said they preferred nettle relief – even with the stings – to their usual drugs, and seventeen said they'd continue with it. Nettles work just as well inside you, too, especially for gout victims: they help cleanse irritating wastes from joints. They also supply a mineral, boron, which is especially helpful in arthritis. In one trial, 70% of a group of 1257 arthritic patients showed improvement after taking a daily dose of 1.5g of dried nettle for three weeks.

Here's an idea for you...

When you're stiff and aching all over at the end of a long day take a bedtime ginger bath. To prepare it, peel and slice a three-inch chunk of fresh ginger root into a pan of water, bring to the boil and simmer until it's a strong dark yellow. Add some Epsom salts to enhance the effect. Strain, add to a warm bath and soak in it. Afterwards, do a little gentle stretching, then slip into bed. Ginger boosts circulation to ease inflamed joints

Ayurveda, the traditional medicine of India, draws on medical texts over 1500 years old. The gum resin of the *Boswellia serrata* tree (the source of aromatic frankincense) is mentioned in these texts for its antirheumatic and anti-inflammatory powers, and Indian doctors have been using it ever since. Tests carried out at Indian government research centres have not only shown how effective it is, but have also demonstrated its freedom from such side effects as raised blood pressure or heart rate, ulcers or irritation of the gut which are sadly common with conventional anti-arthritic drugs. Boswellia relief kicks in quite fast: you may notice an improvement in as little as a fortnight.

In Ayurvedic prescriptions for arthritic disorders, boswellia is often combined with turmeric, the spice that gives curries their lovely deep yellow colour. Turmeric contains compounds called curcuminoids which are great inflammation fighters. This spice has been nicknamed the aspirin of India, so widespread is its use in family first aid.

'I've been eating celery ever since we last met,' said a friend of my sister when I went to stay with her recently. I looked blank. 'Remember, I told you about my arthritis, and you advised me to eat lots of celery? Well, that was five years ago, and my arthritis hardly bothers me now,' he said happily. In fact, the whole celery plant is rich in anti-inflammatory compounds. Its seeds are especially potent. They help flush out the tiny pain-causing crystals of uric acid which can build up in joints – classically, the big toe – to cause agonising pain. So eat plenty of celery or celeriac, and drink celery-seed tea.

'We don't believe in rheumatism or true love until we have been attacked by them.'
MARIE VON EBNER-ESCHENBACH, Austrian writer

Defining idea...

Centuries ago, people observed the white willow tree's preference for damp boggy sites, and figured that it might help conditions made worse by damp climates. They were right: an extract of the tree's inner bark effectively reduces pain and inflammation in gout or rheumatoid arthritis. Scientists identified a chemical called salicin as the wonder-working ingredient in willow's make-up: chemically tweaked in the laboratory, this evolved into everyone's favourite painkiller, aspirin. But the downside to aspirin is its irritant effect on the stomach. The salicin in willow may not work as fast as aspirin, but it's kinder to your gut, although you should avoid it if you have a serious gastric problem.

In a 2004 German study, 4731 patients with arthritis or back pain took doses of willow bark over six to eight weeks. Most of them had given up on their non-steroidal anti-inflammatory drugs (NSAIDS) either because they weren't very effective or because of the side effects. By the end of the trial, average pain intensity across the group had fallen from 6.4 to 2.7, with 18% reporting no pain at all, while only 1.3% reported minor side effects. Don't take it, though, if you're on warfarin or aspirin.

Arthritis is a complex condition with any number of possible contributing factors. Consult a medical herbalist who, after taking a detailed medical history, will tailor a herbal prescription for your specific needs and problems.

171

How did it go?

Q I've heard that devil's claw might be good for my rheumatism. Sounds alarming! Should I take it?

A *It's a sprawling plant that grows in the baking hot Kalahari desert of southern Africa. The natives nicknamed it devil's claw on account of the curved barbs on its roots which often maim their cattle, but an extract of its root tubers is now an effective treatment for many joint problems. In clinical research in South Africa, France and Germany, patients have reported relief of pain, increased mobility and general improvement in well-being, with very few side-effects. It doesn't work for everyone, but it is fast-acting when it does: its benefits are usually felt within ten to fourteen days. Don't take it if you are on prescription drugs. Mild gastrointestinal upsets are an occasional side-effect.*

Q Can you suggest a herbal cream I can apply to my sore, aching joints?

A *In a clinical trial, Arnica gel was as effective as ibuprofen at reducing the pain and improving the flexibility of swollen osteoarthritic hands. Use it on any joint – especially last thing at night, so that they're less stiff on waking. However, don't use it on broken skin. Herbalist Dee Atkinson invites her patients to use cabbage poultices on inflamed joints, especially knee joints. Take a rolling pin, she instructs them, across the veins in the cabbage leaf and then bandage it round the joint. Add some heat via a hot wheat bag or a hot water bottle, and leave the poultice on all night. This can give a lot of relief.*

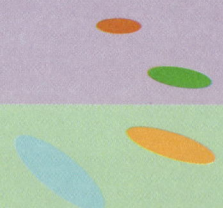

172

41

Pains, strains, sprains

Ouch! You just pulled a muscle, strained a tendon or sprained an ankle.

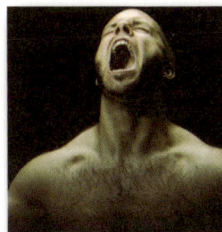

It happens all the time to footballers, rugby players, cricketers — and they're out of action for weeks on end.

But most of us can't take that kind of time off, or afford all that intensive physiotherapy. We need something to ease the pain fast, and get us going again. Try a little herbal relief.

Two great herbs, arnica and comfrey, head the first-aid list.

Arnica – a gorgeous little yellow flower which grows in high mountain meadows – has been used for centuries by country people to treat bruises, sprains, strains, swelling and fractures, and calm the pain that they cause. It's a marvellous remedy to keep on hand in your first-aid kit. You can buy it as a cream, but the gel is easier to apply. And it's so effective at relieving joint pain that when researchers tested it on the stiff, swollen hands of osteoarthritis patients in a clinical trial comparing it with ibuprofen, the arnica gel produced by a Swiss company was rated every bit as good. Arnica is powerful medicine, however, which should never be taken internally, or used on broken skin. Some people, especially pale-skinned redheads, can have a irritated skin reaction to it, so do a patch test before you use it. The same

Here's an idea for you...

My family swears by a wonderful French aromatherapy product, formulated by Dr Valnet, which works wonders for stiff, sore or aching joints and muscles. Stiff neck, a spot of back pain, achy calf-muscles from overdoing the aerobics? Out it comes, giving unfailing relief every time. The key ingredient is ginger, a powerful anti-inflammatory which speeds up the local circulation to relieve pain or swelling. Try a ginger bath: add 2–3 teaspoons of powdered ginger to a pint of hot water and simmer till it turns yellow. Then add it to your bedtime bath.

Swiss company have produced an arnica bath oil, adding a little wintergreen, to soak your aches away. Wintergreen is another great plant remedy for pain and inflammation, which turns up in a lot of liniments and massage creams for sports injuries.

Country names for herbal remedies often tell you what they were good for. In the case of comfrey – a tall rough hairy plant with big leaves – its various names leave you in no doubt at all: knitbone, knitback, bruisewort, boneset. It does in fact contain a substance called allantoin that speeds the healing of bone and tissue by upping cell proliferation. Comfrey has been valued for centuries as an unparalleled remedy for wounds, cuts, sprains, aches of every kind. It can be used in the form of creams, oils, ointments, hot infusions of the dried leaves applied as compresses or simply the fresh green leaves pounded and used as a poultice. (Don't take it internally, though.)

German-born herbalists Peter and Barbara Theiss also recommend a comfrey root paste as 'the best kind of treatment for all types of traumatic damage to bones, tendons, and muscles... such as fractures, bruises, sprains, strains, contusions'. To make the paste, they instruct, put 3–4 heaped tablespoonfuls of the powdered root in a bowl and add enough hot water, plus a little vegetable oil, to stir it into a paste. Apply it as hot as bearable to the affected area, cover it with a piece of cotton, bandage it into place and leave it for several hours or overnight. Then remove the compress and massage with comfrey ointment. I can't imagine why this wonderful herb isn't used more often.

'Sprain: tearing or stretching of the ligaments that hold together the bone-ends in a joint, caused by a sudden pull.'
The British Medical Association's *Complete Family Health Encyclopedia*

Defining idea...

The essential oil of lavender offers wonderful relief for sore, stiff and aching muscles, soothing pain and reducing inflammation. Add 5–6 drops of the oil to a teaspoonful of almond oil and stroke it into the affected muscles.

If you have a nasty fall, resulting in a severe strain and bruising, the pain can be acute. If it's likely to linger on, try one of the great herbal anti-inflammatories, which can be so valuable for rheumatism but which take a little time to kick in. Devil's claw, boswellia and white willow are three to look for: they all have established reputations in the treatment of arthritic ailments. Take them in pill or tincture form from a reliable herb supplier, and follow the directions on the label.

How did it go?

Q   **My boyfriend does quite a lot of sport, and somebody told him that tiger balm was brilliant for sorting out the odd muscle aches and stiffness he often suffers from. What is this stuff exactly?**

A   *Tiger balm was developed centuries ago by Chinese herbalists as a soothing ointment for aches and pains. It contains aromatic herbs, spices and essential oils chosen for their pain-calming powers – menthol, camphor, clove and cinnamon among them. The recipe was perfected by a nineteenth-century Chinese herbalist, Aw Chu Kin, whose son launched it on the market. It's fantastic stuff; you can almost see it getting the local circulation going. Your boyfriend needs the red version, which is specific for muscle pains. Don't worry – no tigers are sacrificed to make it!*

Q   **I get terrible leg cramps, usually in the middle of the night when the sudden pain wakes me up. What do you suggest?**

A   *You may be deficient in important minerals; magnesium particularly, or calcium or potassium. Or you may be dehydrated, so try drinking three or four glasses of water a day above and beyond your usual fluid intake, and see if matters improve. The essential oil of rosemary is wonderfully warming and analgesic. Put 2 drops in a teaspoon of almond or olive oil and massage it into the affected leg just before you go to bed, stroking it gently upwards, and make sure you're warm enough in bed.*

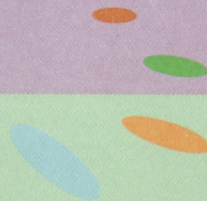

42

The baby herbal

Babies respond very rapidly to both herbal and orthodox medicines.

This means that even the gentlest of herbal remedies can have a remarkable effect.

There's no need for complex and costly herb remedies either. You can treat most of your baby's problems from a very small range of herbs – many of them available as tea bags.

Stock your herbal medicine chest with chamomile, elderflower, limeflower and catnip tea bags; a small bottle of almond oil; bottles of the essential oils of lavender, neroli and chamomile; small bottles of comfrey and St John's wort oil; and marigold, comfrey and chickweed creams or ointments. Babies and toddlers need much smaller doses of herbal tea than grown-ups. Give a baby just a dessertspoonful in a little tepid boiled water, and a tablespoonful or so for a toddler.

A baby who can't sleep becomes a problem for the whole family, exhausted by broken nights. To help babies sleep peacefully, put three or four tea bags of chamomile or limeflower in a jug of boiling water and infuse, covered, for ten minutes, then add to baby's bedtime bath. Or add 2 drops of lavender, chamomile

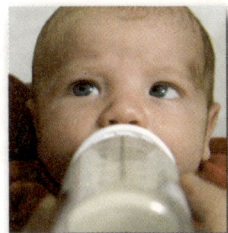

Here's an idea for you...

Your doctor will assure you that cradle cap is quite harmless. But if it really bothers you, add 2 drops of lavender oil to 2 tablespoons of olive oil, and rub it gently into your baby's scalp at bedtime. In the morning, gently shampoo off the loosened crusts.

or neroli essential oil to a cup of whole milk, stir well and add that to the bath instead. Some babies love to be stroked: give them a bedtime massage on their back or feet with a teaspoon of almond oil to which you add a drop of lavender oil. If the baby keeps waking up, make up a cupful of chamomile tea, and put a dessertspoonful in a bottle with some tepid boiled water. A drop of lavender oil on the pillow also encourages sleep.

Colic in babies can be caused by wind, sensitivity to milk and dairy products or, if you are breastfeeding, that chicken vindaloo you enjoyed last night. If a baby is already on solids, it could be something he or she ate. If the baby is breastfed, suggests herbalist Dee Atkinson, the trick is to get mum to drink a nursing tea. She makes one up for her patients that contains fenugreek, peppermint, raspberry leaf, fennel, chamomile and dill – all soothing, calming, antispasmodic herbs. They are passed on to the baby through breast milk; the tea, incidentally, tastes delicious! If the baby is bottle fed, fennel or dill seeds are soothing for tiny colicky stomachs: put half a teaspoon of either in a cup, fill with boiling water and infuse, covered, for ten minutes. Then strain it, let the liquid cool and give teaspoon doses. Chamomile tea works well, too.

Babies can get really bad nappy rash, sometimes caused by irritant chemicals in the nappy wash. Fresh air and, if possible, sunshine are the best cure. Between nappies, leave your baby's bottom bare for as long as possible. Before you put baby back into a clean nappy, wash his or her bottom with very diluted marigold lotion, dry very thoroughly, and apply one of the following: comfrey cream or oil, marigold cream or chickweed cream. For a change, you can also try zinc and castor oil ointment, with a little of one of these mixed with it.

Teething? Give your baby a liquorice stick or a long piece of marshmallow root to chew on, or rub the gums with diluted marigold lotion. At bedtime, give chamomile or catnip tea to help a teething baby sleep.

It sometimes happens, even in the best of families, that a baby is born. This is not necessarily cause for alarm.
ELINOR GOULDING SMITH, humorist and writer

Defining idea...

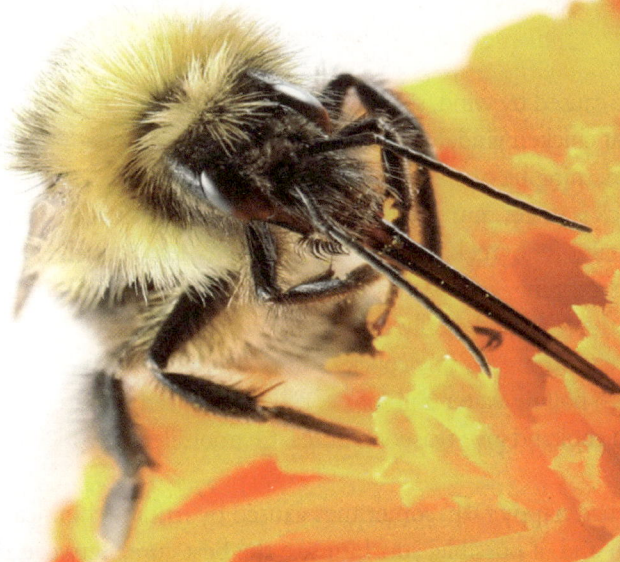

How did it go?

Q   Our nine-month-old baby has two or three times run a temperature and looked quite hot and restless. My wife always panics and wants to rush her to the doctor. Is this really necessary?

A   From time to time babies will suddenly spring a fever on you. But baby temperatures fluctuate much more readily then adults', so unless she seems especially distressed, simply put her to bed with a warm herbal infusion of elderflowers – which have mild antiviral activity – or chamomile or lemon balm three times a day. Give her plenty to drink: plain bottled water or diluted organic fruit and vegetable drinks. Carrot is especially helpful. If she's very warm and restless, give her a tepid sponge-down but cover her up immediately afterwards and don't let her get chilled. However, if her temperature stays high and she seems really miserable, call the doctor. Babies over a year old can be given a dose of echinacea, which will boost their resistance in case of viral infection. Use one of the special formulations for children, and follow the dosage on the label.

Q   Our baby gets really horrid diarrhoea from time to time. What can we do about it, and should we call the doctor?

A   All babies have diarrhoea from time to time but if it persists, and the baby is feverish or in pain, call the doctor at once. For mild cases, give plenty of liquids. Chamomile tea diluted in plenty of tepid water is good, or – a French country remedy – a very thin purée of organic carrots, made by cooking 450g scraped and grated carrots in a litre of boiling water, which is then strained and given in a bottle. If your baby is on solid foods, keep them simple: vegetable purées with a little rice or potato. Avoid fruit until the diarrhoea has cleared up, with two exceptions – grated raw apple purée is especially helpful for upset tummies, and so is mashed banana with a touch of cinnamon.

43

Herbal healing for kids

The commonest children's ailments are mild fevers, coughs, colds, sore throats, upset tummies and problems getting to sleep.

In my experience, they can usually be treated successfully from a very small range of mild but effective herbal remedies.

Save antibiotics for real emergencies. If you use herbal remedies instead of the constant doses of paracetamol or courses of antibiotics so many parents seem to rely on, you'll help your children build their own natural resistance.

Coughs, chesty colds and sore throats crop up regularly even in the healthiest children. But even if your child develops an alarming fever, a nasty cough or a lingering sore throat, and you decide to visit the doctor, you can still begin immediate treatment with doses of an echinacea specially formulated for children, as well as drinks of elderflower tea or doses of elderberry syrup, both great immune-system boosters with antiviral clout into the bargain.

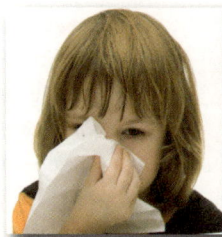

Here's an idea for you...

Children often develop the pink itchy eyes of conjunctivitis. To treat it, make up a cup of chamomile tea, let it cool, and gently swab your child's eyes with the tea. Then apply the used – and now cool – tea bag to the affected eye as a compress. Remember that hands must be scrupulously clean when you're touching eyes, and wash them afterwards. Repeat a couple of times, and at bedtime. If the eye isn't better within a day, go to the doctor.

Elderflower makes one of the nicest of herbal teas: use a tea bag and let it infuse, covered, for five minutes. You can sweeten it with a touch of honey; for a bedtime drink, combine the elderflower with a peppermint tea bag in a big mugful of boiling water. Give a small cupful of this – it will help sweat out the cold overnight.

A Russian cough remedy which I used many times for our two daughters is made with two or three fat cloves of garlic. Slice them into a small glass, add a couple of tablespoonfuls of honey and leave overnight, covered with cling film. Give teaspoon doses of the runny liquid that will result three or four times a day.

Too much excitement, too much bedtime television, or just a bright and active mind can all keep children tossing and turning instead of sleeping. A small cup of chamomile tea, with a dot of soothing honey, is often all that's needed. A drop of the essential oil of lavender on the pillow can work wonders, too. And if they're really wound up, use several limeflower tea bags to make a strong infusion, and tip it into a warm bedtime bath.

Upset stomach? Limeflower or chamomile tea will usually do the trick, plus a nice long rest. Give the child plenty of water to drink, as well. If there is nausea, grate a little fresh peeled ginger root into the teacup too, or choose peppermint tea.

Defining idea...

For a sore throat, infuse a sprig of fresh sage (or half a teaspoon of dried) in a cupful of boiling water, covered, for five minutes. Add a dash of vinegar and persuade your child to gargle with it two or three times a day. If he or she hates the taste, put a big dollop of a high-fruit blackcurrant jelly in a cup, add a little lemon juice and pour boiling water over it. When it's cooled, the child can gargle with it two or three times, for as long as possible, then drink what's left. Blackcurrants fight soreness and inflammation, and they're very rich in vitamin C.

Cuts, scrapes, grazes? Use calendula ointment, made from marigold flowers; it takes the ouch out of these with amazing speed. I used the lotion, diluted in a little warm water, to wash the dirt out of grazed knees, treated mild cases of sunburn and applied neat to the painful inflammation that often followed the first ear-piercing.

How did it go?

Q **Our children always seem to be picking up head lice at school. I don't want to use the powerful chemical shampoos the school suggests. Is there anything both safe and effective?**

A *Head lice are increasingly resistant to those strong chemical treatments you worry about. Luckily, there's a much simpler solution now, based on neem, the wonder tree from southern India which has been used for centuries for pest control as well as skin problems, oral hygiene and fungal infections. Head-lice treatment shampoos based on neem have a pleasant, clean smell, are as easy to use as a normal shampoo, can be rinsed out in minutes, and you don't have to ply the nit comb afterwards. So far, there have been no cases of head-lice resistance to neem. You can use tea-tree oil, too.*

Q **Our family holidays have been upset quite a few times now when one of the children develops a nasty ear infection. Do we have to take them to the doctor for antibiotics?**

A *Try these simple herbal remedies first; they'll usually stop the pain and clear up the problem very quickly. Herbalists use a combination of garlic –antiseptic – and mullein, which is analgesic. US herbalist Aviva Romm gives this recipe: put a chopped whole bulb of garlic, 25g of mullein flowers (from any herbal supplier) and 500ml olive oil in a stainless steel or enamel pan, simmer over very low heat for thirty minutes, then strain it into a clean jar and keep in the fridge; it will last up to two years. Warm a little of the oil in a teaspoon over a lighted match, check it's not too hot, and dropper 3–7 drops into the affected ear. Then put a little cotton wool in front, to keep it in place. You can also buy the garlic-mullein oil ready made – a useful holiday standby. If there's a discharge, the pain persists or the child has a high temperature, call the doctor.*

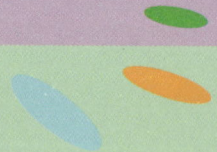

44

The green traveller

Travel sickness, sunburn, hangovers, Spanish tummy, mosquito bites, sleepless nights – who needs them on holiday?

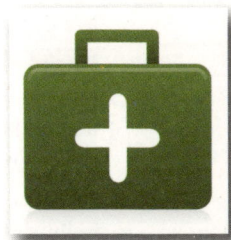

Pack a carefully picked herbal first-aid kit, though, and with any luck you'll have a hassle-free hol with no trips to the local pharmacy to spoil your fun.

For some luckless people, travel itself is the first health hurdle, and motion sickness can turn a car or sea trip into a nightmare. Much the best remedy – and perfectly safe for children – is ginger: take it an hour before the trip starts, and then every two hours or so. The easiest way to take it is in the form of powdered ginger in capsules, or you can grate two inches of peeled fresh root into 300ml of limeflower tea: use two tea bags and infuse for five minutes, covered, in the boiling water, then drink a cupful before you leave. Take the rest in a thermos flask for occasional swigs during the journey (limeflower tea is also soothing for the nervous stomach). Some people find that chewing crystallised ginger does the trick, and I've even known people swear by straight ginger ale.

Here's an idea for you...

When our eighteen-year-old daughter went off to India in her gap year, I gave her a packet of garlic pills and begged her to take one every day. To her (and our) surprise she returned without having suffered a single day of Delhi belly, despite such indiscretions as milk shakes on the beach at Kerala. Garlic is a potent bactericide, working to prevent any infection starting up in your gut – and beefing up your immune defences into the bargain.

If you or your children dread travelling by plane – quite a common problem – pack some of Dr Bach's Rescue Remedy in your hand-baggage: this mix of flower essences is fantastically effective at calming apprehension, panic, terror. On a flight some time ago, I sat next to a woman who before take-off was shaking and literally white with terror; I gave her some Rescue Remedy, and she calmed down enough to relax for the rest of the flight. Air travel, incidentally, can leave your skin completely dehydrated so pack a tiny spray bottle filled with your favourite flower water for use on the plane. Rose would be a great choice.

Unwashed fruit or salads, contaminated shellfish, dodgy meat, too many chemicals in the cheap local vino, even the local drinking water (and the ice made from it in your gin and tonic): any of these can bring on the cramps, the nausea and the misery of travellers' diarrhoea. I never travel without a herbal remedy based on tormentil, which is a little yellow-flowered weed remarkably high in tannins. These astringent chemicals work to calm diarrhoea by reducing inflammation in your inflamed and irritated gut. Prickly brambles supply another popular old country diarrhoea remedy – the thin bark of blackberry roots is also rich in tannins, and even the fruit has been known to work. There are tannins in common tea, too, but as a diarrhoea remedy, drink it black. Green tea is even better.

Grated raw apples are a common country cure for diarrhoea: pectin, the soluble fibre in apples, helps soak up toxins and soothe the gut. Drink plenty of water, meanwhile; preferably bottled. If the diarrhoea isn't any better after a couple of days – especially in the case of small children – or if there's blood in your stool, seek medical help.

> '**No man needs a vacation so much as the man who has just had one.**'
> ELBERT HUBBARD, American editor, publisher and writer

Defining idea...

Holiday hell is the whine of bloodthirsty mosquitoes during a hot and sleepless night. If your bedroom isn't mosquito-proofed, you'll need to wear an effective repellent. I dislike deet-based ones and my favourite is a natural, delicious-smelling moisturiser called Alfresco. It contains a range of essential oils formulated by a clever lady who once worked at London's Chelsea Physic Garden and passed rigorous testing at the London School of Tropical Medicine. Numbers of film stars working in bug-ridden locations have sworn by it – including Mel Gibson when filming *Braveheart* in the midge-ridden moors of Scotland.

The essential oil of lavender works both as repellent and bite-soother: a few drops on your pillow, or in a burner beside your bed, will repel the mozzies as well as helping you sleep, and you can apply it neat to bites and stings. (That bottle of lavender oil should be wrapped up tight in cling film before packing, by the way, unless you want your entire holiday wardrobe to smell of lavender.)

Hangover? Go back to your favourite bar the morning after, and ask the sympathetic barman for a tot of Fernet Branca, an Italian liquor based on a wide range of digestive herbs, and a tried-and-tested hangover remedy.

How did it go?

Q **We're off to Bali for our holiday next year, and I'm already dreading the jet lag. Can you suggest any solutions?**

A *Soviet cosmonauts used Siberian ginseng, the great stress remedy, to help them adjust to the ravages of space travel. Take it for three days before travelling, and continue until three days after your arrival. When you get there, go to bed and get up at the local time, no matter what time of day you arrive.*

Q **I always seem to end up with sunburn on holidays however careful I am. How can I deal with it?**

A *Take a fat tube of aloe vera gel. The cost of that glorious tan is often two or three nights of sunburn agony. The moment you realise you've overdone it, step into a cool shower and stay there as long as possible. Then towel off and apply aloe vera gel all over the sunburnt bits. It's the single best remedy for sunburn I know. Failing that, lavender essential oil can be applied neat to badly burned areas.*

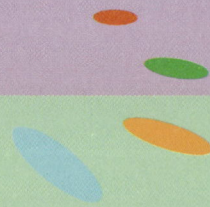

45

Pets in peak form

If you use herbal remedies yourself, why not try them for your pets too? They're gentle, they're cheap and they're wonderfully effective.

Some of the herbs in your own first-aid kit work just as well for dogs and cats.

Your garden or kitchen will provide a wealth of wonderful food medicines you can use – parsley, dandelion, nettles and watercress among them. With a handful of safe and simple remedies you can see your pet through a number of health problems. Of course you'll need to consult your vet if your pet is injured or seriously ill, but even then herbs can help soothe pain, speed up healing and calm nerviness or fear.

Healthy pets won't need much doctoring, and healthy means properly fed. 'Ask any holistically minded vet, and they'll tell you: it has been very noticeable that skin, digestive and behavioural problems have all increased dramatically since those complete dry foods became so popular.' That is Mary Boughton speaking and she should know; her parents founded a British company over fifty years ago making licensed herbal medicines for animals, and she's worked with animals all her life. 'Many of these commercial dried foods contain synthetic colourings and flavourings to make them look more attractive, and they put a huge strain on the kidneys,' she explains. Feed your pets fresh, natural and unprocessed food as far as possible.

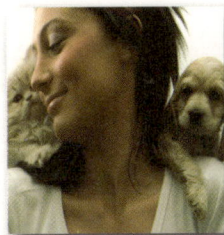

Here's an idea for you...

Give your pet his daily greens! Finely chopped or puréed dandelion leaves, watercress, spinach or parsley are all wonderful food medicines and mineral-rich dietary supplements, to be added in teaspoon-sized doses to your pet's feed. Purée a quantity at a time, fill an ice-cube tray with them and freeze. Defrost a cube or two as needed.

If you give your pets only one herb make it garlic. It boosts their resistance to infections by strengthening the immune system, cleanses the whole system and helps repel any kind of parasites. A regular daily dose will help protect them from infections and viruses such as kennel cough. You can buy garlic tablets that are especially formulated for dogs and cats, with dosage-per-size directions which you should observe.

Fleas are a perennial irritation (in every sense of the word) for pets and their owners. Careful, regular grooming to remove fleas is vital for successful prevention. Dogs should be washed with a gentle herbal shampoo and Mary suggests one containing pennyroyal, which repels fleas without any risk of irritating a pet's sensitive skin. Before country walks, dust them with powdered neem leaf, specially on those vulnerable hairless bits. Keep baskets or kennels clean, and strew them with herbs whose strong odour will make fleas think twice before moving in. Try dried rosemary, mint, lavender, sage, wormwood, southernwood or pennyroyal.

Itchy skin? Suspect an allergic origin; if your pet lives on dry processed food, he could be reacting to additives in it. For immediate relief, there's no better remedy than common or garden nettles. In spring or summer, gather tender young nettle tops, purée them and add to the day's feed, adjusting the dose according to your pet's size – starting with a coffeespoonful for small pets. Otherwise, sneak a little dried nettle into your pet's feed.

190

Diarrhoea? Fast your pet for a day, and then give him a teaspoonful of slippery elm powder mixed with enough water to make a liquid. Once swallowed, the slippery elm will turn into a soft jelly which calms and heals an irritated gut. If the diarrhoea persists, consult your vet.

There's one herbal medicine that dogs always rush to nibble: the tough couchgrass which makes them heave and vomit minutes later. Don't ever stop them: Juliette de Bairacli-Levy calls it 'an admirable intestinal cleansing herb'. It's your dog's very own year-round detox. For a more thoroughgoing one, you can buy special detox pills formulated for dogs, with cleansing peppermint and parsley among their ingredients. They're specially formulated not only to remove toxins from the system, but also to neutralise that antisocial doggy reek that comes from an unhappy gut.

Sooner or later the most active pets can slow down and show signs of stiffness or pain in moving. Make sure their diet is super-healthy, complete with the omega-3 essential fatty acids found in freshly ground linseed or cod liver oil. Mary Boughton recommends a daily dose of celery seeds: 'very effective in reducing arthritic and rheumatic pain'. Soak them in warm water for a day, she suggests, then add to the feed.

By the way, don't experiment: pets are not people. Some of the most effective herbal medicines for humans have never been tested on animals, and may actually harm them. Echinacea, for instance, has been known to damage canine immune systems. And aspirin is fatal to cats, so don't give them willow or meadowsweet.

'...it rests in the hands of the human owners as to whether an animal is to live its full life span in true and total health, or to be cut off by disease in early infanthood, or to live a miserable life of subhealth.'
JULIETTE DE BAIRACLI LEVY: *The Complete Herbal Handbook for the Dog and Cat*

Defining idea...

191

How did it go?

Q **I dread the fireworks season – my poor King Charles spaniel tries to dig himself into the carpet with terror when the big bangs start going off. Can herbs help?**

A *Well, valerian is a sedative for the nerves which works wonders to calm them down. So does that other great soother, skullcap, and you can buy special veterinary tablets in which these two herbs are combined. For desperate cases, try the Bach Flower Remedy Rock Rose – it's especially for terror! Add a couple of drops to your pet's bowl of drinking water. Cats don't usually react as badly, but most cats will calm down at a mere sniff of valerian.*

Q **We use marigold all the time in my family. Is it safe to use it for pets if they have bites or cuts?**

A *Definitely. If your pet is badly bitten, your vet needs to check there's no serious damage needing attention. But for lesser injuries, soothe calendula oil onto the affected spot. Or add a teaspoonful of the tincture to some warm water, soak a strip of towelling with it and apply as a comforting compress. Keep it in place as long as your pet allows, and renew it from time to time.*

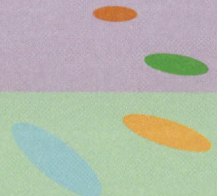

46

The herbal spa

Soaking in a hot scented bath is one of the nicest ways to unwind.

Add the right herbs or essential oils, and it can also be a tonic for the spirit, a terrific beauty treatment and a wonderful remedy for a wide range of human woes.

Your skin is porous, so soaking in a bath containing herbal infusions or essential oils is a very gentle way to absorb their medicinal properties. Indeed, in the case of essential oils, it's one of the best ways, along with massage, since they should never be taken internally except under expert direction.

As a general rule, a herbal spa bath should be pleasantly warm rather than hot, especially during the day. Save hot baths for bedtime, when they can relax you and soothe aching muscles. Their effect will be enhanced if you give yourself a quick cool-to-tepid shower at the end, or – if your bath has no shower attachment – pull the plug out, run in plenty of cold water, and have a quick splash in the cooling water.

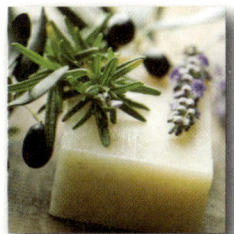

Here's an idea for you...

If you have plenty of nettles in your garden, enjoy a nettle bath: great for arthritis, sunburn, aching muscles or even inflamed and itchy eczema. To make it, put a couple of generous handfuls of nettles in a big pan, pour over 2 litres of boiling water. Simmer for five minutes then take off the heat and infuse for another ten minutes. Strain the liquid and add it to your bath; keep it warm rather than hot.

Very hot baths can be debilitating, and are an especially bad idea if you suffer from high blood pressure, a heart condition or varicose veins. Essential oils, incidentally, evaporate very rapidly in high temperatures. Make your own personal blend of essential oils for a luxury bath. Rose, geranium, ylang-ylang, neroli and lavender are all particularly lovely, uplifting smells.

Water, paradoxically, is drying to the skin. Add oatmeal to your bath, and it not only soothes and moisturises – a beauty secret known to the ancient Egyptians, the Greeks and the Romans – but it's also a well known treatment for the irritated itchy skin of eczema sufferers. You can buy the specially finely milled colloidal oatmeal, which can be added straight to the bath. Or you can use ordinary oatmeal: simply stuff a cupful into the foot of a pair of clean tights, knot it over the hot tap, and a creamy liquid will flow out into your bath when you run the water. To enhance the soothing effect of oatmeal, add 5–10 drops of lavender or geranium essential oil.

Another terrific skin-softener is apple cider vinegar. You can make up your own herbal bath vinegar by half-filling a preserving jar with fresh herbs, then filling it right up with cider vinegar, closing it tightly and leaving it in a dark place to infuse for three to four weeks. Then strain it through a coffee filter paper and put it in a clean stoppered jar: don't forget to label it or it might turn up in your salad dressing! The herbs need to be absolutely clean and dry. Choose rosemary for a wonderful morning pick-me-up, peppermint or ordinary garden mint for a great refresher (perhaps before you go out in the evening), thyme if you're feeling out of sorts and chesty, lavender flowers to soothe muscle aches, balm to calm your spirits and chamomile or marjoram to help you wind down at bedtime.

'There must be quite a few things that a hot bath won't cure, but I don't know many of them.'
SYLVIA PLATH, *The Bell Jar*

Defining idea...

Health-food stores and supermarkets these days stock a huge range of herbs, both single and mixed, in handy tea-bag form, so brew up a strong infusion, using four to five bags at a time, and tip it into your bath.

No time for a therapeutic bath? Try soaking up the herbal remedy via your feet. If you've been rushing or, worse still, standing around all day and your feet are killing you, soak them for ten minutes in a warm footbath to which you have added 4–5 drops of peppermint essential oil or a mug of very strong peppermint tea; use three tea bags. When you get that achy, chilly, coming-down-with-a-cold feeling, give yourself a bedtime footbath of limeflower and elderflower – a strong infusion, half a cup of the fresh herbs each to a good litre of boiling water, infused covered and then added to the footbath. You could use two tea bags of each, well-brewed.

How did it go?

Q **I read somewhere that a hot footbath can help see off a headache. Is this right?**

A   *Yes, it can: make the footbath very hot, soak your feet in it for ten minutes, then plunge them into cold water. It's even more effective if you make a strong infusion of rosemary – pour 500ml of boiling water over 3–4 sprigs of rosemary and infuse, covered, for ten minutes before straining the liquid and adding it to the footbath.*

Q **I often add essential oils to my bath but 5–6 drops doesn't seem to make much difference. Should I use more than this?**

A   *I discussed this with Marie-Therese Tiphaigne whose French company produces organic essential oils, and who worked very closely for years with Dr Jean Valnet, the founding father of modern aromatherapy. She makes two points. First, that it is very important to add the oils to a dispersing base – her company produces its own excellent one – before adding them to the bath water. If you don't do this, they can collect on the surface and some of them can be quite caustic when in contact with the skin. If you have no dispersing oil at hand, she suggests half a cup of milk, but it must be whole milk. Secondly, for a therapeutic effect, she suggests around 20 drops in total, though no more than 10 of the following oils: thyme, oregano and savoury. Pregnant women, incidentally, should only use camomile, geranium, lavender or rose, and then only 3–4 drops.*

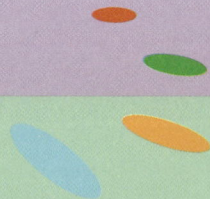

47

Grow your own

Create your own green pharmacy. If you have a garden, a patio, a balcony – or no more than a wide windowsill – you can grow herbs to treat a whole range of minor ailments.

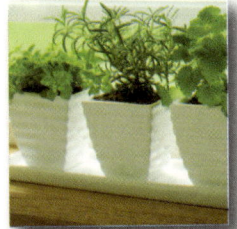

Most of them will add zest and flavour to soups, stews and salads, too.

If you have green fingers and room to spare, plant a miniature herb garden with all your favourites. If you're a hopeless gardener, or if space is limited, buy plants in pots in the spring, and transplant them into larger pots, with more good compost, as they grow. Better still, plant them out straight away – two or three at a time, into big pots – to give yourself a plentiful supply. You can order beautiful organic plants online, and some supermarkets sell them too.

Herbs like plenty of sunshine: think of the hills of Provence, fragrant with the smell of thyme, rosemary and marjoram. Water them regularly, and treat them to some good natural fertiliser from time to time. (The dark liquid I tap off from my wormery from time to time is a fantastic growth-promoter.) Finally, site them as near your kitchen as possible; in a downpour, you don't want a long trek to the thyme.

Here's an idea for you...

To add colour to your herb garden, fill a big pot with nasturtiums – wonderfully easy to grow. These dazzling edible flowers are high in antioxidants, with mild antibiotic powers into the bargain. Add them to salads as a gentle boost to your immune system.

Start with the classics. Thyme, with its strong pungent scent, is a wonderful antiseptic: make an infusion, using 3–4 sprigs to a cupful of boiling water, and drink it for coughs, colds, sore throats, general chestiness, asthma. Or if you have a whole bush of it, you can make a really strong brew, simmering a big mugful of the fresh herb in a litre of water, covered, for twenty minutes, then tip it into a bedtime bath.

Like thyme, sage is powerfully antiseptic: especially for any infection or inflammation of the mouth and throat, gargling repeatedly with an infusion of the herb leaves will often clear up the problem almost overnight. Traditionally, it can help boost a flagging memory – a small clinical study confirmed this recently. Sage also helps dry up secretions of all kinds, so although nursing mothers must avoid it, it's a boon to menopausal women, who find that an infusion of sage drunk cold can ease the misery of hot flushes.

I'd always want lemon balm with its sweet lemony smell in my herb garden: tea made from the fresh leaves is incomparably better than the dried version. Lemon balm is one of nature's soothers: drink an infusion to calm indigestion, stomach cramps, menstrual pains, general nerviness. It's mild enough for children too: a great 'goodnight' herb. You need plenty for your cuppa: at least three teaspoons of the fresh leaves to a cupful of boiling water. And, as with all herbs, infuse it covered.

In Morocco, early morning sees the mint vendors appear at street corners, their little carts loaded with the fragrant bright green mint which will be stuffed into teapots and glasses for every Moroccan's favourite cuppa: mint tea. They make it with green tea, plenty of the variety of mint called *Mentha spicata*, and a lot of sugar – but almost any of the dazzling variety of mints will do. Nicholas Culpeper, a particularly savvy English herbalist, claimed that mint was 'useful in all disorders of the stomach', so try it for gripes, cramps, spasms, nervous 'butterflies' in the stomach. It's also worth a try for morning sickness, and give children a little honey-sweetened mint tea to sip when their tummy hurts. To make it, put a small bunch of the fresh leaves in a mug, fill it with boiling water, cover and infuse for five minutes, then strain and drink. And don't forget the mint sauce when you enjoy hard-to-digest roast lamb; the Ancient Romans also made mint sauce for pork, for fish – and for 'wild sheep'.

Down the centuries, rosemary has had an awesome reputation, both among doctors and in folk medicine, for its power to boost both memory and general alertness. What's certain is that it's a great tonic to kick-start a busy day and a marvellous pick-me-up when you're feeling dog-tired at the day's end, or at moments of great stress or fatigue. To make rosemary tea, put three or four of the fresh green tops in a mug, fill with boiling water, cover and infuse for ten minutes, then strain and drink with a little honey. A rosemary bath is a great way to start the day, too: dump a couple of handfuls of rosemary in a stainless steel pan, fill with cold water, bring to the boil and simmer, covered, for twenty minutes. Strain and add to your bath.

'Why should a man die who has sage growing in his garden?'
Popular medieval saying

Defining idea…

199

How did it go?

Q **I have just bought a garden flat, and the end of the garden is full of nettles and dandelions. What can I do with them?**

A *Lucky you! Cherish them both. Nettles are an excellent natural mineral supplement, rich in the iron, calcium and silica needed for strong bones and shiny hair. They help the body flush out the excess uric acid responsible for gout, and nettle tea is an old folk remedy for rheumatism. Drink it, too, for hay fever, or if your skin breaks out in an allergic rash. And harvest the tender young tops to add to soups and casseroles, or cook like spinach. Dandelion is the king of liver tonics: add the young leaves to salads, soups or steamed vegetables for a wonderful fillip to your whole digestive system.*

Q **I love the scent of lavender, but can you actually take it internally?**

A *Definitely: it's one of the great stress-busting herbs, relaxing to mind and body; take lavender tea for headaches, hangovers, anxiety, stress or sleeplessness. But it's quite powerful, so I usually add just a pinch of the flowery tops to a cup of chamomile or limeflower tea.*

48

Soothing storms with a teacup

The herbal infusion known simply as tea is drunk all over the planet for its pleasant stimulating effect, but plenty of other herbs make great teas too...

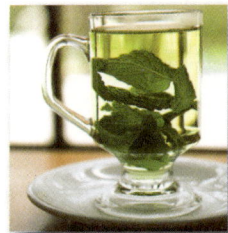

Discover some of nature's rich variety.

There's an ever-growing demand for herb teas, and you can buy a dizzying variety in tea-bag form. You can also buy a number of great herbs in combinations aimed at specific problems such as stress, respiratory or skin ailments and general detox. Buy the herbs loose, though, and store them away from light, in labelled jars, and you'll find they have a fresher, more vivid taste as teas. You can use more than the often rather stingy amounts in tea bags, and you can also experiment and develop your own personal blends.

Keep a glass or china teapot specially for your herb teas, make them with the loose herbs, and pour them out through a strainer, just as we all used to do before tea bags were invented. Teapots are a good idea, since most herb teas should be infused covered.

How much herb to use? For a single cup or mug, a good teaspoonful of dried herb; more if it's fresh. And infuse for a good five to ten minutes. If you're using roots or bark, they need to be simmered (in a stainless steel or enamel pan, please) for about ten minutes to draw out their goodness.

Here's an idea for you...

When I was living in Italy, some friends of ours in the country served this aromatic tisane as a digestive after a summery lunch. Take 2 sprigs of thyme, 2 of mint and 10 rose petals – any colour will do. Pour 2 cups of boiling water over them and leave them to infuse, covered, for three to four minutes. Then strain and serve.

The black tea we all love is rich in antioxidants; green tea is even more so, though if you like your tea with milk, it loses that antioxidant punch. But some of the best-known herbs taste so good they can be drunk on their own. Chamomile, the great calmer, has a warm, mellow, slightly apple-y flavour. Limeflowers and elderflowers both have a gorgeous smell of summer. Peppermint is, well, minty. Lemon verbena – another gentle calmer of nerves and stomach – has a clean, fresh lemony taste, as does lemon balm, a cheery, uplifting tea.

I combine three of these in a lovely after-dinner tea: one part limeflower, one part lemon verbena, and – if you have it – a few fresh lemon balm leaves. It's a warm, citrussy, aromatic brew, and a great substitute for coffee.

Many valuable herbs taste, frankly, boring – grassy, hay-like, bland, earthy or just sort of green. So if there are serious medical reasons for choosing a particular herb, and its taste doesn't thrill you, you can always blend it with a herb that has real zing. Nettle tea, for instance, is so mineral-rich it's better than any pill, and a great calmer of allergic problems into the bargain, but you might as well drink an infusion of spinach. Mix it with zesty, minty peppermint, though, and it slips down a treat. If, like me, you find green tea both bland and slightly bitter, copy the

Moroccans who get through gallons of their favourite mint tea: green tea brewed in silver teapots with sugar and plenty of the fresh herb – marvellous for the digestion.

Here are some other ways to zizz up teas. Add a scrap of lemon or orange peel, a pinch of cinnamon or ginger and, for sweetness, a little honey or a pinch of powdered stevia if you can find it; it's sweeter than sugar and actually good for you.

When herbalist Alex Martin came to lunch with me, she brought me one of the special teas she mixes up for her patients, with names like Blues and Flus, Revitalise and Wake Up. Her choice for me was Tranquillity, now one of my favourite bedtime drinks: it's made with two parts each of limeflower and chamomile, and half a part of lavender. 'Limeflower soothes the nerves,' she explained. 'Chamomile helps digestion, and lavender helps you sleep – but lavender is a very up-front taste, so you don't need too much of it.'

If you have specific health problems, match your tisane to your personal needs. Nerves, depression, anxiety? Try lemon verbena, chamomile, lemon balm. Respiratory problems? Limeflower, elderflower, ginger, thyme. Troubled skin? Red clover – a mellow, delicate flavour – nettle, marigold. Digestive problems? Meadowsweet, peppermint, ginger, fennel seeds. Need a general tonic? Sage or rosemary.

'Thank God for tea! What would the world do without tea? How did it exist? I am glad I was not born before tea.'
SYDNEY SMITH

Defining idea...

203

How did it go?

Q **My local coffee bar is offering something called 'Chai Tea' these days. Sounds intriguing. What exactly is it?**

A *Chai tea is a lovely, warming, spicy brew, perfect for a cold winter day. The Indians, who invented it, are as addicted to it as we are to our mid-morning coffee. The spices in it boost circulation, aid digestion, and help keep colds at bay. To make it, put a teaspoon of grated fresh ginger, 3 peppercorns, half a cinnamon stick, 4 cloves, 12 cardamom seeds, a curl of orange peel and a pint of water in a pan. Bring to the boil, cover and simmer for ten minutes. Add half a cup of whole milk, and honey or brown sugar to taste, and bring it back to the boil. Add 3 teaspoons of loose black tea, take off the heat and let it infuse for three minutes. Then strain, pour and enjoy.*

Q **I get a lot of colds and respiratory problems every winter. Can you suggest a tea I could drink as protection?**

A *I asked Croatian herbalist Dragana Vilinac to suggest a nice warming protective tea for you. Here's her suggestion. Stock up on dried elderberries and echinacea root from a herbal supplier, keep fresh ginger on hand, and you can drink it throughout the long dark days of winter. Great for convalescents, too, says Dragana. To make the tea, put 5g of elderberries, 5g of echinacea root and 5g of grated fresh ginger root in a pan, cover with a mugful of water, bring to the boil and simmer, covered, for ten minutes. Strain it and add a little honey before drinking.*

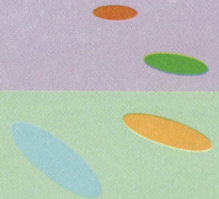

49

Good hair days

You can't be beautiful without beautiful hair, said a famous shampoo ad, and it's hard to disagree.

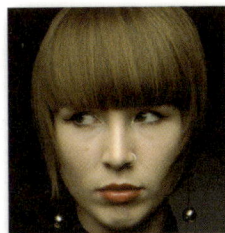

No matter how good your looks, or eye-catching your outfit, sad, limp, lifeless hair will always let you down.

This is why women – not to mention film stars, celebrity footballers and cricketers – spend fortunes at the hairdressers and beauty counters. Throughout history, dozens of plants have been used in the pursuit of those lustrous locks. Many of them perform quite as well as clever modern chemicals, so if you hate the idea of soaking your head in synthetics, go for these natural beautifiers. Some of them could be growing in your own garden and numbers of these star in the various 'green' all-natural cosmetic ranges.

Good circulation in the scalp is critical for hair health. Whenever you shampoo your hair, give your scalp a mini-massage. Tense your fingers as though you were clutching a tennis ball, and hold the scalp firmly while you make gentle rotating movements all over your head. Rosemary is a great circulation booster: try adding 5ml of the essential oil to 100ml of vodka, and using it as a scalp friction. If your hair is looking tired, choose a rosemary shampoo, or make a strong infusion of rosemary, and use it for the final rinse.

Here's an idea for you...

Bone-dry, lifeless hair? Give it the oil treatment, using one of a quartet of great oils to nourish and revive your hair. Choose from the jojoba oil beloved of Mexican women, the sesame oil of the Far East, the coconut oil of the tropics or the olive oil which gives Mediterranean women their wonderful glossy hair. Warm the oil first, then apply it to dry hair and scalp, combing it through your hair to the tips. Massage your scalp for five minutes, then wrap a warm towel round your hair and leave as long as possible – at least thirty minutes. Then apply neat shampoo to the scalp, massage it in and rinse off.

The snowy shoulders of dandruff are a real turn-off. Cider vinegar will usually get rid of it fast. Before you shampoo, mix one part of cider vinegar with one part of water, pour it onto your head and massage your scalp for about five minutes. Add a good splash of cider vinegar in the final rinse water, too; that's good for even healthy hair. Dandruff can result from a fungal infection, so add a teaspoonful of tea-tree or neem oil to a bottle of your ordinary shampoo to help clear it.

To speed the process, make a strong infusion of peppermint, thyme, bay or rosemary – a good bunch in a basin of boiling water, then infused, covered, for ten minutes. Cool and apply this to your hair and scalp; leave it on for as long as possible before shampooing.

If your hair is greasy, that daily shampooing is really bad news: it simply encourages the overproduction of sebum. To correct this, put a tablespoonful of dried lemon balm, yarrow, marigold, horsetail, peppermint or rosemary in a glass jar. Add 500ml of cider vinegar, close the jar and leave the mixture to macerate for two to three weeks. Then strain out the herbs, dilute with a little water, and use a couple of tablespoonfuls in the final rinse.

Long before modern chemical hair-dyes were invented, women were using plants to enhance their hair colour. They're no match for modern hair colourings, and they won't last for weeks, but they'll be a lot better for your hair.

'Gorgeous hair is the best revenge.'
IVANA TRUMP

Defining idea...

Whichever herb you use, make a strong infusion using a good handful of the fresh or dried herb – or three to four tea bags where appropriate – in 400ml of water. Use it as a rinse, leaving it on as long as possible. Use camomile or bright yellow mullein flowers for fair hair, elder leaves, nettles, rosemary or sage for dark hair, and sage and rosemary for grey hair. Redheads can treat themselves to a henna colouring, a terrific nourishing treat for hair.

Excess levels of a male hormone has been linked with hair loss in both men and women. In clinical studies, nettle root has been shown to inhibit production of this hormone. Steep a handful of the roots (you can order them from a herbal supplier) in 500ml of cider vinegar, as above, and use it, first, for a regular scalp friction, and then in the final rinse. Dilute the vinegar with equal parts of water. Treat your hair from the inside too: drink nettle tea (you can buy it in tea bags). Nettles are particularly rich in minerals, including silicon, vital for hair health. For a great hair tonic, boil up a good handful of nettles in a litre of water, strain the nettles out and rinse the liquid through your hair.

Almost all shampoos contain highly alkaline detergents which can strip out natural oils secreted by glands in hair follicles to give hair its bounce and sheen. Shampoo no more than twice a week, and use one of the 'green' shampoos in which minimal detergent is balanced by protective oils.

207

How did it go?

Q **I've tried all kinds of oil treatments but my hair still looks very dry. I there anything else I can do?**

A *Hair needs nourishment from inside, so if you want a gorgeous head of hair, eat a healthy diet with plenty of vitamin E and the essential fatty acids found in fish oils or linseeds (also known as flaxseeds), and all the B-complex vitamins. Make sure you get plenty of the antioxidants found in brightly coloured fruit and vegetables. And a regular supply of sulphur, please – that's found in onions, watercress, cabbage, horseradish – because sulphur is a key ingredient in hair health.*

Q **I've heard that Frenchwomen use nasturtium to treat their hair. What does it do?**

A *French herbalists recommend sulphur-rich nasturtiums for every kind of hair problem including weak, thinning hair or hair loss. If you have them in your garden, pick a handful of the leaves and the bright yellow and orange flowers, simmer in 400ml water for twenty minutes, then strain and use for the final rinse. Eat the flowers in summer salads, too!*

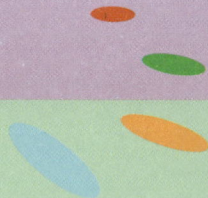

50

Great skin

It's fashionable to be green – and when it comes to skin care, it might even be life-saving.

Do you really want to risk your health for the sake of a flawless face?

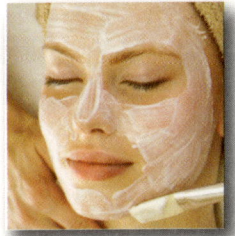

It's been calculated that women who use make-up on a daily basis are absorbing almost 2.25kg of chemicals a year through their skin. Most of those prettily packaged creams and lotions are a cocktail of dozens of chemicals, including fragrances, preservatives, artificial colourings and mineral oil. Some are irritants which can trigger eczema or dermatitis, some are carcinogenic, some cause genetic mutations, and others can disrupt our hormonal, nervous and immune systems. And when US researchers studied thirty-three brand-name lipsticks, they found that three in five of them also contained lead – a very potent brain poison.

So declare your bathroom a chemical-free zone, and stock up on skincare products based as far as possible on plants, fruits and essential oils.

There are a growing number of 'green and natural' skincare ranges on the market, some of them organic, made using a minimum of synthetic chemicals, if any. And some of the best and most effective skin treatments – flower waters, natural oils, herbs – don't even need clever formulation, just a reliable supplier.

Here's an idea for you...

Need a quick pick-me-up for greasy or dull-looking skin? Make up some peppermint tea, using just half a cup of boiling water to a tea bag. Cool it with ice cubes, then spritz it onto your face.

Long before the cosmetic industry invented itself, women the world over were using natural oils from local plants both to cleanse and nourish their skins – jojoba and coconut, olive and avocado among them. These oils work to peel off dirt, dead cells and old make-up while preserving the skin's natural acid mantle which protects and lubricates it. They're also filled with natural antioxidants, to counter the free-radical activity which can age and damage skin, and essential fatty acids to feed your skin. Just film a tiny amount of your chosen oil all over your face and very gently massage it in. Leave it for a couple of minutes – or while you soak in a bath – then remove with damp cotton wool. It will leave your skin clean, smooth and moist, and needing no extra moisturiser. Choose the best-quality cold pressed and organic oil, and use it up while it's fresh. For dry, sensitive or ageing skin use almond, sesame, coconut or avocado oil; for normal skin, olive or jojoba, and for greasy or problem skin, sunflower or coconut oil.

Two exceptional oils, to apply to freshly cleaned skin, and both fairly new to the Western market, are argan oil from Morocco and *Rosa mosqueta* oil, from the hips of a wild Chilean rose. Argan oil has been used for centuries by Moroccan women to rehydrate ageing or sun-dried skin, or to treat skin scarred by acne or chickenpox. *Rosa mosqueta* is building itself a dazzling reputation for its ability to reduce scarring, wrinkles and sun spots, and improve the skin's natural elasticity. In a fascinating trial carried out by two Chilean skin specialists, twenty women aged between twenty and thirty-five who spent summers at the beach were given *Rosa mosqueta* and asked to apply it daily from May to August. Despite their sun exposure, surface wrinkles smoothed and sun spots almost disappeared. By the end of the trial, the faces of the women still looked smooth and fresh.

Apple cider vinegar leaves skin soft and smooth. Add a good splash of it to a basin of cold water and rinse your face in it for a wonderful morning reviver. You can turn it into a customised beauty treatment by steeping herbs in it. Put a big handful of clean, dry and fresh herbs, or 30g of dried herb, in a large preserving jar. Cover with a litre of apple cider vinegar, seal and store in a dark place for three to four weeks, then strain off into a clean stoppered jar and label it carefully. Marigold flowers, geranium leaves, lavender, chamomile flowers, lemon balm or limeflowers all make lovely vinegars.

'The skin is, or should be, the expression of one's good health, so if you want to help nature a little by caring for your skin, use nothing but biological cosmetics, especially those of natural plant origin, since they stimulate and support the skin's natural functions. Other cosmetics are little more than paint.'
ALFRED VOGEL, *The Nature Doctor*

Defining idea...

How did it go?

Q **I know rose water is good for the skin. Are there any other flower waters?**

A *Flower waters, or hydrolats, are a by-product of the distillation of essential oils, and are becoming more and more popular. They are also a cheaper way to enjoy your favourite essential oils – geranium, jasmine, ylang-ylang, for instance. Try lavender for oily or problem skin, orange flower water for dry or mature skin, and elderflower, which is mildly astringent and stimulant. Aromatherapist Carolyn Marshall uses hydrolats all the time in her practice: 'I give my clients little 10ml atomisers filled with their favourite, to spray onto their skin as a wonderful morning freshener. I use a lot of Helichrysum, commonly known as eternal flower: it's marvellous for dry, itchy or inflamed skin, or to soothe the itchy blisters and crusts of chickenpox.'*

Q **I've heard that steaming is good for the skin. Mine is quite greasy – can you give me some suggestions and help?**

A *A herbal steam is a nice pick-me up for any skin type. For you, I'd suggest marigold flowers, nettles or peppermint. Dry skins? Parsley or violet, and lemon balm or limeflower for normal skin. Here's how you do it. Put two big tablespoons of the dried herbs – more if they're fresh from your garden – in a deep glass or china bowl and cover with two litres of boiling water. Give them a stir, then wrap a towel round your head and the basin. Bend over – not too close or you'll scald yourself – and give your face a ten-minute steam while you listen to some nice music. Then strain and cool the liquid, use it to rinse your face and finish with a splash of cool water.*

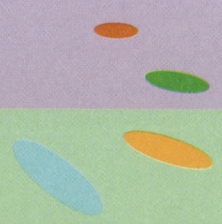

212

51
Nice footwork

Be good to your feet: they work their socks off for you.

If you value your comfort, think of theirs.

Don't cram your feet into ill-fitting shoes, keep tottery high heels for party best, avoid sweaty synthetic socks and footwear. Wash your feet thoroughly at least once a day, and if your job keeps you sitting or standing around for hours on end, give them a little extra pampering at the end of it.

For tired, overworked feet, herbalists Peter and Barbara Theiss recommend a warm footbath and a short plunge in cold water at bedtime, then a gentle massage with calendula ointment (made from marigolds). 'Every time', they report in their book *The Family Herbal*, 'we find that they are refreshed and fully recovered by the next morning.' Peppermint is another great refresher. If you have some of the essential oil, add 5 drops to a warm footbath and give your feet a good soaking. You can also use a couple of tea bags to brew up a strong infusion: add it to that warm footbath. Follow either with a quick cold splash.

If young Christopher Dean hadn't picked up a severe infection in a toenail thirty years ago, tea-tree oil might not be so widely popular today. After five months of treatment, the London School of Tropical Medicine declared the infection incurable, with surgery the only option. At which point his brother arrived from Australia with a small sample of tea-tree oil and suggested he give it a try. Within ten minutes the pain eased, within four hours the swelling subsided, within four days his feet were normal. Christopher went back to Australia to help found the first tea-tree oil company, and today it has an annual turnover of over $20 million.

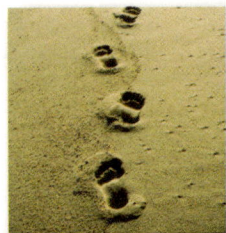

Here's an idea for you...

Next time you get a nasty big blister on your heel or toes, resist the urge to pop it and risk a nasty infection. Instead, dab it as often as possible with distilled extract of witch hazel. It will dry out the blister and relieve the pain, too. Once it has flattened, apply marigold cream on a plaster to speed the healing process.

Tea-tree oil is still the first choice for obstinate bacterial or fungal infections affecting your feet. After a thorough wash, dry off your feet and paint the oil directly onto the affected bits. Do this last thing at night. Keep your feet dry, wear cotton socks and shoes made of natural fabrics so that your feet can breathe. Fungi just love the warm, moist sweaty atmosphere of trainers and nylon or acrylic socks.

If the infection persists, alternate the tea-tree oil treatment with footbaths of thyme or sage. To make them, put a handful of the fresh herb, or a good tablespoonful of the dried, in a stainless steel or enamel saucepan, fill it with water, bring to the boil and simmer, covered, for twenty minutes. Then strain, add the liquid to a warm footbath and soak your feet for ten minutes. Use it up within a day.

You can combine the sage or thyme treatment with apple cider vinegar – one of the great folk cure-all remedies, popular for centuries. To do this, put a bunch of fresh sage or thyme into a stainless steel or enamel pan, add two cups of the vinegar and then simmer, covered, for fifteen minutes. Strain, add a good dash to a warm footbath, and soak the feet two to three times a day. Dry your feet thoroughly before pulling on socks.

Yet another great plant antiseptic, oil from the neem tree, can work wonders with athlete's foot. Paint the oil onto the infected bits at night; in the morning, wash and dry your feet thoroughly, then dust powdered neem between the toes.

'When our feet hurt, our bodies hurt.'
SOCRATES

Defining idea...

There are hundreds of traditional corn cures. Try this one from Greece: paint the corn with lemon juice and tape a piece of lemon peel on overnight. Onion juice is another country favourite. And a great skin softener is castor oil (don't drink it!) – cover the corn with a ringed corn plaster, and apply a drop of castor oil two to three times a day.

A friend of mine told me that her schoolboy son was desperate because the verrucas on his feet were not just hurting, they were keeping him out of the swimming pool; he'd been having treatment for weeks without success. I gave her a tube of green clay and a small bottle of tea-tree oil. 'Add a drop to a teaspoonful of the clay paste and apply it to the wart,' I suggested. The verrucas cleared up almost overnight.

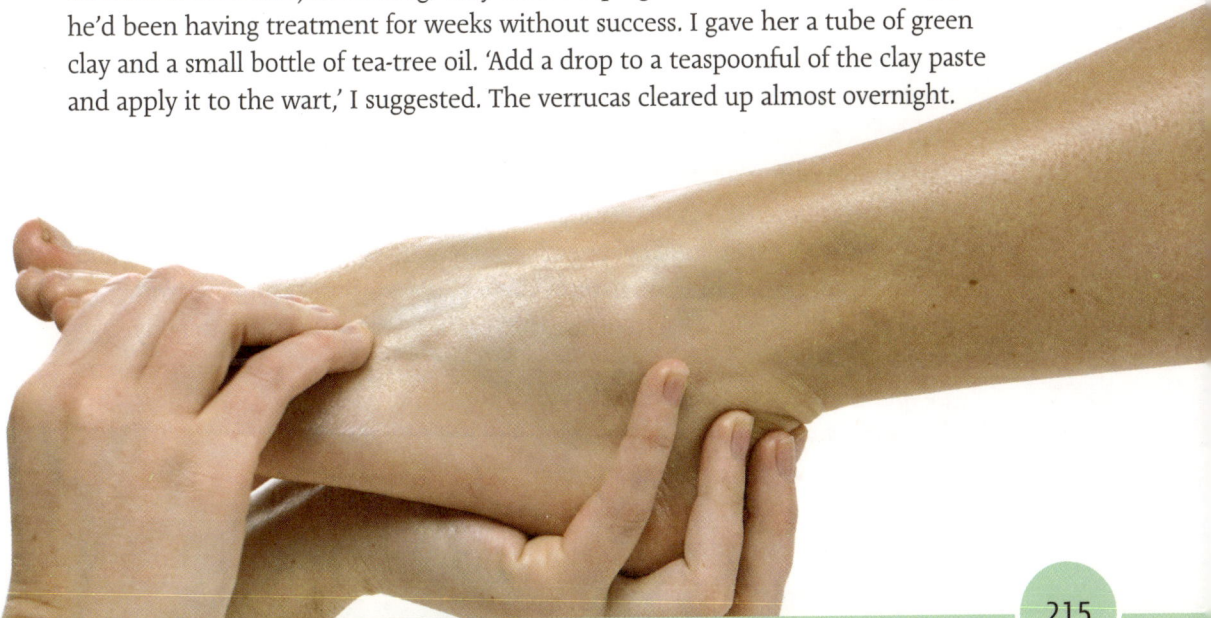

How did it go?

Q **My partner has desperately smelly feet. They don't seem to worry him much but he's willing to follow suggestions up to a point. What do you think might work?**

A *Persuade him to take a warm footbath once a day, to which you add 5 drops of cypress essential oil – a nice manly smell, very popular in aftershaves. Its astringent action will help keep his feet dry and deodorised. As a morning splash, treat him to a bottle of either sage or cypress hydrosol: this is the water produced when essential oils are distilled. Finally, dust neem powder into his shoes.*

Q **Every winter I suffer agonies from chilblains. What can I do about them?**

A *Try a country remedy: mix cayenne pepper half and half with talc and sprinkle it in your socks. Australian herbalist Robyn Kirby points out that chilblains result from poor circulation, and recommends a general tonic made up from tinctures of three herbs that all help boost it. Mix 100ml of prickly ash with 100ml of ginger, then add 10–20 drops of cayenne. Take half a teaspoonful three times a day. With this tonic, says Robyn in her book Herbs for Healing, 'I have cured forever the tendency to chilblains of many, many patients.' To ease the agony, you could also try this blend of essential oils suggested by aromatherapist Franzesca Watson in her book Aromatherapy Blends and Remedies: 6 drops of rosemary, 3 drops of peppermint, 3 drops of lavender. Add these to a 30g jar of aqueous cream from the chemist, stir well and soothe it into the chilblains night and morning.*

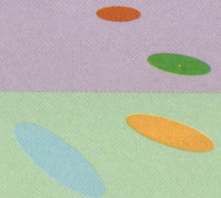

52

The family medicine chest

For most minor ailments, the family medicine chest is the first port of call.

Stock it with a chosen number of herbal remedies and you'll find yourself coping effectively with any minor medical crisis that happens along.

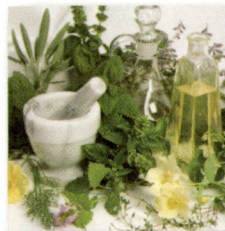

Over the years I have got to know herbs that can deal with cuts and grazes, bumps and lumps, colds, sore throats and flu, burns and scalds, aches and pains, hangovers and upset tummies, viral infections, earache and toothache. In my experience, they are just as effective as the alternatives and, as some of them are marvellous multitaskers, I find they often work out cheaper too.

Marigold
If I could take just one herbal remedy to a desert island, it would have to be the amazing marigold, often called *calendula*, one of nature's premier healers. It soothes pain, counters inflammation, speeds healing. I use the tincture, diluted, as a comforting lotion for burns and scalds; to heal over acne pustules which the sufferer couldn't resist picking open; as a comforting wash for the pain of shingles; as a healing disinfectant for cuts, grazes and small infections, such as those in newly pierced ears; and as a remedy for toothache and gum infections (soak a small swab

Here's an idea for you...

Collywobbles after that curry dinner? Touch of food poisoning? Bad case of the runs? I keep on hand a Swiss-made extract of the little yellow-flowered wild plant tormentil, which has exceptional binding powers in the gut. Relief is usually fast – though if disagreeable symptoms persist, see a doctor.

of cotton wool with it, and place next to the infected tooth or gum, keeping it there for several hours). The ointment, smeared on a plaster, stops the pain of a cut or infected sore, treats wounds of any kind, calms the agony of piles, and soothes reddened baby bottoms.

Lavender

The essential oil of lavender is another herbal multitasker. I dab it neat on mosquito bites and it works as a repellent, too. I add 8–10 drops to a warm bath to help me feel calm and relaxed, apply it neat to minor burns or scalds once I've cooled them with cold water, and put 1–3 drops on the pillow of a baby, restless toddler or insomniac adult to encourage sleep.

Arnica

Arnica gel is powerful stuff for bruises and swelling, muscular aches and pains, and the stiff sore joints of arthritis. In a clinical trial, a Swiss-made arnica gel proved itself an anti-inflammatory as effective as ibuprofen when applied to swollen arthritic joints. (Don't apply it to cut, irritated or broken skin, though.)

Comfrey

Comfrey cream, ointment or oil is marvellous first aid for cuts and messy grazes. It also helps prevent nasty bruising after a fall, and should be stroked gently into sprained or strained muscles or fractured joints. It's a rapid healer of both flesh and bone because of its power to boost cell-proliferation. Like arnica, it's not to be taken internally.

Aloe vera

Every home should have a tube of aloe vera gel: it's marvellous first aid for burns, scalds, sunburn and itchy or irritated skin. It can even help cool the agonising inflammation of shingles.

'*Our kitchen cupboards, our gardens and our hedgerows are full of potent medicines for almost every common ailment.*'
ANNE MCINTYRE, *The Top 100 Herbal Remedies*

Defining idea...

Mullein

If there are children in the house, keep a little dropper bottle of mullein oil. It has for centuries been a popular country cure for earache, usually combined with garlic. Dropper it into the affected ear at the first symptom of heat and pain.

Propolis

Cold sore? You can already feel it tingling in your upper lip. Zap it with a couple of drops of the tincture of propolis, a sticky resin manufactured by bees and used in the construction of their hives. Propolis is a specialist in mouth problems. Apply it neat, with a cotton-wool bud, to mouth ulcers; it will tingle for a moment. Add 8–10 drops to a little warm water and gargle several times daily to see off a sore throat.

Blends

In our family we also swear by a French blend of essential oils in a base of tincture of ginger, formulated by Dr Valnet, the founding father of modern aromatherapy. This pale golden aromatic lotion is a magical calmer of aches and pains when gently massaged into aching muscles, stressed backs or tired joints. Another great Valnet formula combines essential oils that work to sort out respiratory problems. Containing pine, mint and lavender among others, it smells like a walk through a pine forest. You spray it on a hanky – or on your pillow at night – to inhale it, or put it into a burner, all to ward off or treat colds.

How did it go?

Q   **There are lots of herbal teas on the shelves of my local supermarket. Are these OK as herbal remedies?**

A   *In some cases, but not all of them have enough of the herb to constitute an effective dose. And I'd always look for an organically grown herb too. Here are some ways to use them. Try chamomile tea to soothe colic or sleeplessness in babies and small children; as a disinfectant wash for eye infections; as a general soother or calmer. Use the cooled tea bag as a compress for reddened, itchy or sore eyes. Peppermint is the perfect after-dinner drink, great for the digestion; try a stronger brew to add to a footbath for tired, aching feet. Limeflower tea can calm nausea – try it for morning sickness too. Delicious elderflower is mildly antiviral, and is traditionally combined with peppermint and yarrow to stop an oncoming cold.*

Q   **I know that ginger is sometimes used medicinally. Can you tell me more about how I can use it?**

A   *Fresh ginger root can be grated into a mug, topped with boiling water and infused for ten minutes to make a hot winter tea – add a little honey. I also keep a little bottle of ginger juice syrup in my medicine chest. It can be added to a hot whisky toddy to ward off a cold and to a glass of warm water to pacify the pangs of indigestion or settle a nauseous stomach.*

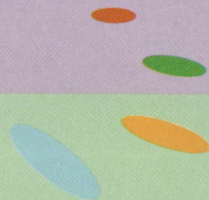

Resources

Many of the products mentioned are available from good health-food stores. If you draw a blank at your local one, the following companies are all reliable suppliers of many forms of herbal medicines, including single herbs, either dried or powdered, in pill, capsule or tincture form. Other products are also to be found in their ranges: essential oils, macerated oils and flower waters. Many supply excellent ready-made combinations of herbs formulated by professional herbalists, and aimed at specific problems such as stress, sleeplessness or detox. These are especially useful if you're not very experienced in the use of herbs. Almost all these companies have websites from which you can order directly, as well as telephone order lines. And most of them will be happy to send you their printed catalogues which are often extremely informative and helpful.

General herbal suppliers

G. BALDWIN & CO.
www.baldwins.co.uk
Mail order: 020 7703 5550
The oldest-established herbal suppliers in the UK: their enormous range includes a comprehensive list of herbs in dried or tincture form or pills or capsules; essential oils and burners, aromatherapy roll-ons, tea bags, creams, ointments and flower remedies.

BEE VITAL
www.beevitalpropolis.com
Mail order: 0845 458 1655
A mine of information about propolis and a huge range of propolis products, including tinctures, tablets, toothpaste and mouthwash.

A.VOGEL
www.avogel.co.uk
Mail order: 0800 085 0820
Bioforce market the superb range of herbal remedies developed by Alfred Vogel, the renowned Swiss naturopath, each made from whole, fresh, unadulterated plants within twenty-four hours of harvesting. The range includes arnica gel and bath oil, Tormentil Complex for diarrhoea, passionflower combined with oats in their Passiflora Complex for stress and sleeplessness, papayaforce echinacea in several different forms, and a range of neem products.

BIO-HEALTH LTD
www.bio-health.co.uk
Mail order no: 01634 290115
An excellent range of dried herbs in capsules and plant ointments.

DORWEST HERBS
www.dorwest.com
Mail order: 0870 7337272
An excellent range of licensed herbal veterinary medicines.

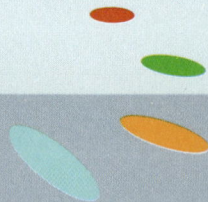

HERBS HANDS HEALING LTD
www.herbshandshealing.co.uk.
Mail order: 0845 345 3727 / International +44 (0) 1379 608201
A comprehensive range of carefully formulated herbal blends for specific health problems, oils, ointments, massage blends, and made-up teas, including Lift and Calm tea, great for hangovers. They also supply Dr Richard Schulze's Superfood Plus.

HIGHER NATURE LTD
www.highernature.co.uk
Mail order: 0800 458 4747
Nutritional and herbal supplements, including Sambucol, the anti-flu elderberry extract, plus a special kids' version, and virgin coconut oil.

NAPIER'S
www.napiers.net
Mail order: 0131 343 3292
A comprehensive range of excellent herbal formulas, some from the company's Victorian founder Duncan Napier – including his famous Nerve Debility Tonic – and others from its modern director, herbalist Dee Atkinson, as well as a huge range of dried herbs and tinctures, mullein-oil formula for earache, and a number of teas, the meadowsweet tea for ulcers among them, and ginger juice syrup.

NEAL'S YARD REMEDIES
www.nealsyardremedies.com
Mail order: 0845 2623145
The largest range of organic skincare and herbal remedies in the UK, available in one of their many beautiful shops or online or mail order. Special baby range, both

Bach and Bush Flower Essences. Full aromatherapy range including organic base oils, remedies to roll, burners. They have blends of teas and tinctures aimed at specific problems, such as a cleansing dandelion and burdock tea, or the buchu and marshmallow tea for cystitis.

THE NUTRICENTRE
www.nutricentre.com
Mail order: 0207 436 5122
The Nutricentre stocks a huge array of health and herbal products, including some of the excellent Planetary Formulas collection formulated by US herbalist Michael Tierra: Kudzu Complex is one of these. They also supply virgin coconut oil and green clay in powder or tubes.

OSHADHI LTD
www.oshadhi.co.uk
Mail order: 01223 242242
A huge range of organic and wildcrafted organic essential oils, flower waters, macerates and carrier oils.

POTTER'S HERBAL MEDICINES
www.pottersherbal.co.uk
Mail order: 0191 370 9466
An excellent range of herbal remedies formulated by professional herbalists.

PUKKA HERBS LTD
www.pukkaherbs.com
Mail order: 0845 375 1744
Some of the most important herbal products from Ayurveda, the traditional medicine of India, including ashwaganda, shatavari, gotu kola and gymnema powder.

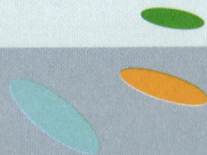

REVITAL
www.revital.co.uk
Mail order: 0800 252 875
Huge range of herbal and other natural medicine products, including HayMax Balm anti-pollen barrier cream, Dr Theiss Swedish Bitters Elixir, and the Natural by Nature aromatherapy range.

RIO HEALTH DIRECT
www.riohealth.co.uk
Mail order: 01273 570987
Rio Health specialises in South American herbal products, including catuaba, guarana, miura puama, maca root and *Rosa mosqueta* oil.

SOLGAR VITAMINS AND HERBS
www.solgarvitamins.co.uk
Stockist enquiries: 01442 890355
Solgar produce an excellent range of herbs in capsule form, including ginger, feverfew, ginkgo, ginseng and the *Scutellaria baicalensis* which many hay-fever sufferers find useful.

VIRIDIAN NUTRITION LTD
www.viridian-nutrition.com
Mail order: 01327 878050
A supremely ethical company, who annually donate 50% of available profits to environmental charities. They have an excellent range of organic herbal tinctures and herbs in capsules.

WELEDA UK LTD
www.weleda.co.uk
Mail order: 0115 9448222
A huge range of herbal products for health and skincare, including bath milks, massage blends and ointments, deodorants, my favourite calendula lotion and ointment, and their new birch juice and elixir. Their herbs are grown biodynamically.

XYNERGY HEALTH PRODUCTS
www.xynergy.co.uk
Mail order: 0845 6585858
Lots of herbal products, including aloe vera gel, the full neem oil range from the Neem Team, ManukaCare 18 honey for wound dressing; the Comvita range of propolis products; and the small but excellent range of herbal products from Kiwiherb in New Zealand, including liquid extracts of echinacea or chamomile specially formulated for children.

Other products

BUTTERBUR FOR MIGRAINES
Linpharma Butterbur Petasin is the only butterbur product on the UK market which is guaranteed to contain at least 15% petasins and is free of pyrrolizidine alkaloids.
Available from:
Natural Figure
www.naturalfigure.co.uk
Mail order: 01506 847 040

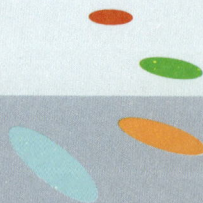

HERBAL TEAS

Dr Stuart's herbal teas, including those served in a London prison to help inmates sleep, are formulated by trained herbalist Dr Malcolm Stuart and can be found in good health-food stores. For more information, visit www.drstuarts.com

NATURAL MOSQUITO REPELLENT

Alfresco is a deet-free natural moisturiser containing botanical extracts of geranium, lavender and melissa, which effectively repels bug, midges, mosquitoes and smells delightful into the bargain.
Alfresco Limited
www.alfresco.com
Mail order: 0208 348 6704

SWISS HERBAL TONIC

Bio-Strath Elixir is a Swiss herbal yeast tonic which, in numbers of clinical trials, has been shown to enhance memory and concentration, increase energy and endurance and strengthen immune function. It's available at good health stores.

VALNET AROMATHERAPY

Dr Jean Valnet's full range of essential oils and aromatherapy products, including Tegarome, Flexarome and Climarome, are available from:
John Bell & Croyden
50–54 Wigmore Street
London, W1U 2AU
Tel: 020 7935 5555

'Green' skincare

Many of the other suppliers have excellent natural skincare ranges, but here are some specialists. There is also a growing number of small companies producing organic skincare: the Soil Association has now certified over 1000 products in this field. These are products of which between 70% and 95% of the ingredients must have been organically grown.

BAREFOOT BOTANICALS LTD
www.barefoot-botanicals.com
Mail order: 0870 220 2273
A range of 100% natural skincare products, with organic essential oils and herbal extracts.

THE GREEN PEOPLE COMPANY LTD
www.greenpeople.co.uk
Mail order: 01403 740 350
Natural and organic skin, body, hair, beauty and baby care products, sun lotions, health and cleaning product for men, women, children and babies

ORIGINS ORGANICS
www.origins.co.uk
A new organic range of skin, body and haircare products, just launched by this well-known US company, and certified not only by the Soil Association, but also by the USDA National Organic Programme, and the French equivalent Ecocert. Visit their website to locate your nearest stockist.

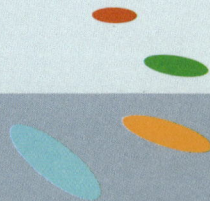

SPIEZIA ORGANICS
www.spieziaorganics.com
Mail order: 0870 850 885
This Cornwall-based family business was founded by an Italian doctor/herbalist and
his wife: many of its beautiful products – made from herbs, plants and oils – are
100% organic, and specially aimed at sensitive skins. The range includes room
fragrances, herbal ointments and skincare.

Suggested reading

Some of the books on this list are out of print, or may be difficult to obtain, even on
Amazon. A very useful website is www.abebooks.co.uk, which specialises in second-
hand books, many of them in as-new condition.

Boughton, Mary: *Herbal Medicine for Dogs*, Amberwood Publishing, 2004.
Buchman, Dian Dincin: *Herbal medicine*, The Herb Society/Rider, 1983.
Chevallier, Andrew: *Menopause*, Amberwood Publishing, 2001.
Conway, Peter: *Tree Medicine*, Piatkus, 2001.
Davies, Jill Rosemary: *The Complete Home Guide to Herbs, Natural Healing, and Nutrition*,
    The Crossing Press, 2003.
Davis, Patricia: *Aromatherapy: An A-Z*, C W Daniel, 1995.
Duke, James: *The Green Pharmacy*, Rodale Press, 1997.
Griggs, Barbara: *Green Pharmacy: The History and Evolution of Western Herbal Medicine*,
    Healing Arts Press, 1997.
Hoffmann, David: *The New Holistic Herbal*, Element Books, 1994.
Kirby, Robyn: *Herbs for Healing*, ABC Books, 1998.
McIntyre, Anne: *The Top 100 Herbal Remedies*, Duncan Baird Publishers, 2006.

– *The Complete Woman's Herbal*, Gaia Books, 1994.
McVicar, Jekka: *New Book of Herbs*, Dorling Kindersley, 2002.
Ody, Penelope: *Essential Guide to Natural Home Remedies*, Kyle Cathie, 2002.
– *Lifting the Spirits: Nature's Remedies for Stress and Relaxation*, Souvenir Press, 2003.
Romm, Aviva Jill: *Naturally Healthy Babies and Children*, Celestial Arts, 2003.
Theiss, Peter and Theiss, Barbara: *The Family Herbal*, Healing Arts Press, 1989.
Tierra, Michael: *The Way of Herbs*, Unity Press, 1990.
Valnet, Jean: *The Practice of Aromatherapy*, C W Daniel, 1980.
White, Linda B., and Foster, Steven: *The Herbal Drugstore*, Rodale Press, 2000.

How to find a herbal practitioner

NATIONAL INSTITUTE OF MEDICAL HERBALISTS
www.nimh.org.uk
Tel: 01392 426022
The oldest and largest body of fully trained medical herbalists in the UK, with members scattered round the world.

COLLEGE OF PRACTITIONERS OF PHYTOTHERAPY
www.phytotherapists.org
This is a smaller body of highly professional herbalists, devoted to achieving the highest standards of scientific rigour in their practice.

THE ASSOCIATION OF MASTER HERBALISTS
www.associationofmasterherbalists.co.uk
Members have a strong affinity with the North American tradition of healing exemplified by the legendary Dr John Christopher.

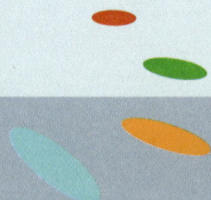

UNIFIED REGISTER OF HERBAL PRACTITIONERS
www.urhp.org
Tel: 07770 782537

REGISTER OF CHINESE HERBAL MEDICINE
www.rchm.co.uk
Tel: 01603 623994
This is a group of over 400 fully trained practitioners of Chinese herbal medicine.
Members do not use any form of endangered animal or plant species in treatment.
'Chinese herbalists' are proliferating in high streets up and down the country but
they are not always staffed by fully trained practitioners, their medicines have not
always passed proper quality control testing and many of them do not speak
enough English to make a thorough consultation possible. If you want to consult a
Chinese herbalist, find one here.

If you would like to learn more about the practice of herbal medicine, there is an
excellent distance-learning course, called 'Discovering Herbal Medicine'. Go to
www.newvitality.org.uk; enquiries to Ms Pamela Bull, course registrar, on 01323
484353. She can be emailed at pamela.bull@btopenworld.com. The course was
originally designed by two eminent herbalists, Hein Zeylstra and Simon Mills, as a
comprehensive introduction to medicinal plants, their properties and uses, to
enable students to make a real difference to the health and well-being of
themselves, their family and friends. It has now been thoroughly updated, and
includes two one-day seminars annually.

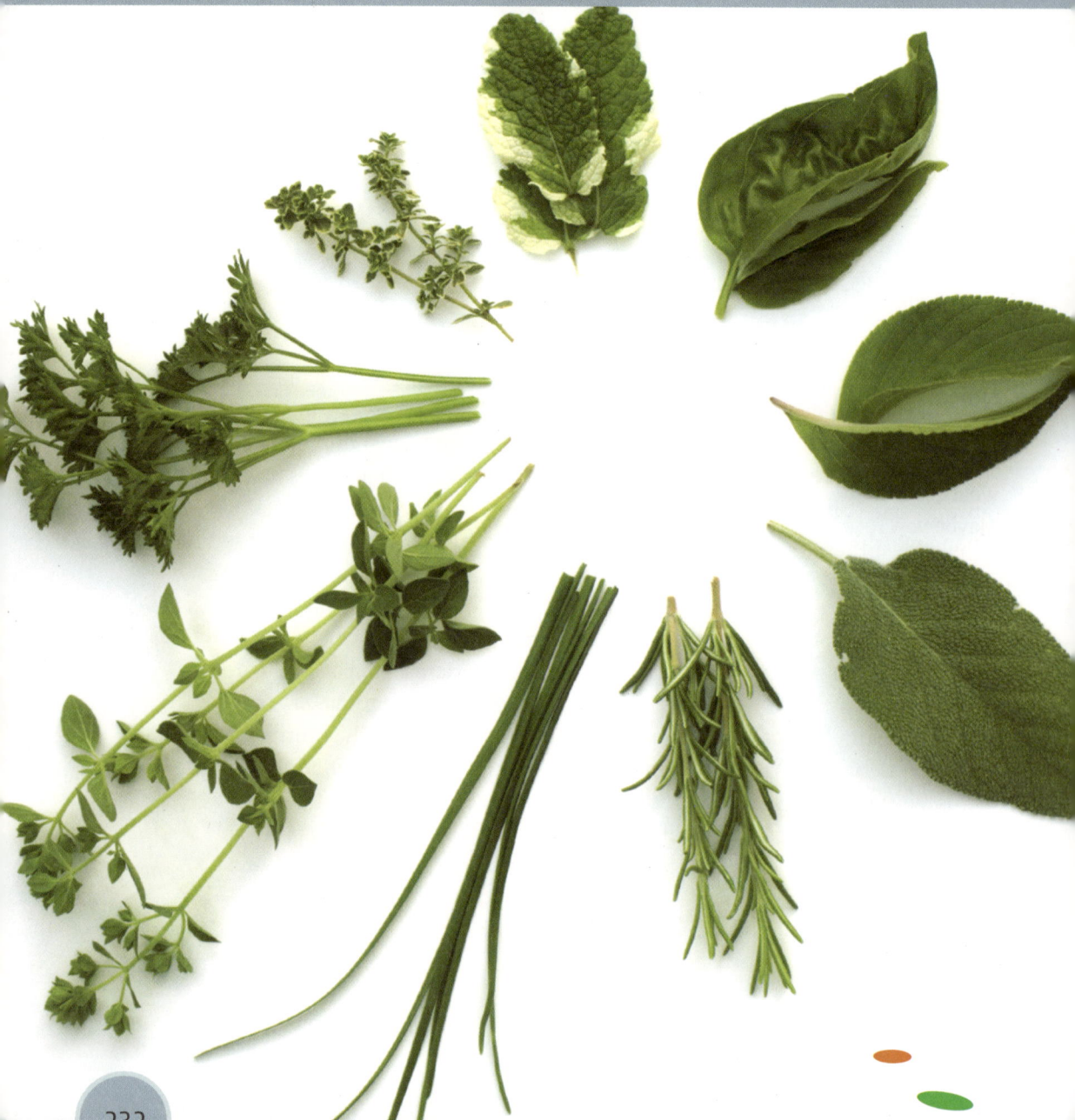

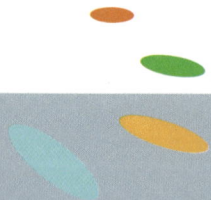

The end...

Or is it a new beginning? We hope that the ideas in this book will have inspired you to try some new things to boost your health, or sort out common ailments. You've added a few essential oils and tinctures to your first aid kit and have maybe even started growing your own herbs. Now you've started using herbs for minor ailments rather than immediately rushing to the pharmacy.

So why not let us know all about it? Tell us how you got on. What did it for you – what really helped you ease the aches, stop the sneezes or get rid of that rash? Maybe you've got some tips of your own you want to share (see next page if so). And if you liked this book you may find we have even more brilliant ideas that could change other areas of your life for the better.

You'll find the Infinite Ideas crew waiting for you online at www.infideas.com.

Or if you prefer to write, then send your letters to:
Helpful herbs for health and beauty
The Infinite Ideas Company Ltd
36 St Giles, Oxford OX1 3LD, United Kingdom

We want to know what you think, because we're all working on making our lives better too. Give us your feedback and you could win a copy of another 52 *Brilliant Ideas* book of your choice. Or maybe get a crack at writing your own.

Good luck. Be brilliant.

Offer one

CASH IN YOUR IDEAS

We hope you enjoy this book. We hope it inspires, amuses, educates and entertains you. But we don't assume that you're a novice, or that this is the first book that you've bought on the subject. You've got ideas of your own. Maybe our author has missed an idea that you use successfully. If so, why not send it to yourauthormissedatrick@infideas.com, and if we like it we'll post it on our bulletin board. Better still, if your idea makes it into print we'll send you four books of your choice or the cash equivalent. You'll be fully credited so that everyone knows you've had another Brilliant Idea.

Offer two

HOW COULD YOU REFUSE?

Amazing discounts on bulk quantities of Infinite Ideas books are available to corporations, professional associations and other organisations.

For details call us on:
+44 (0)1865 514888
Fax: +44 (0)1865 514777
or e-mail: info@infideas.com

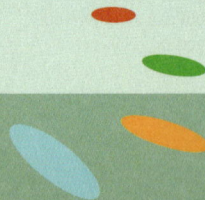

Where it's at...